Current Challenges and New Directions in Preventive Medicine

Editor

MARIE KROUSEL-WOOD

MEDICAL CLINICS
OF NORTH AMERICA

www.medical.theclinics.com

Consulting Editor
JACK ENDE

November 2023 • Volume 107 • Number 6

ELSEVIER

1600 John F. Kennedy Boulevard • Suite 1800 • Philadelphia, Pennsylvania, 19103-2899

http://www.theclinics.com

MEDICAL CLINICS OF NORTH AMERICA Volume 107, Number 6
November 2023 ISSN 0025-7125, ISBN-13: 978-0-443-12989-6

Editor: Taylor Hayes
Developmental Editor: Malvika Shah

Medical Clinics of North America (ISSN 0025-7125) is published bimonthly by Elsevier Inc., 360 Park Avenue South, New York, NY 10010-1710. Months of publication are January, March, May, July, September, and November. Business and editorial offices: 1600 John F. Kennedy Boulevard, Suite 1800, Philadelphia, PA 19103-2899. Periodicals postage paid at New York, NY, and additional mailing offices. Subscription prices are USD $332.00 per year (US individuals), $786.00 per year (US institutions), $100.00 per year (US Students), $416.00 per year (Canadian individuals), $1023.00 per year (Canadian institutions), $200.00 per year for (foreign students), $100.00 per year for (Canadian students), $461.00 per year (foreign individuals), and $1023.00 per year (foreign institutions). To receive student/resident rate, orders must be accompanied by name of affiliated institution, date of term, and the signature of program/residency coordinator on institution letterhead. Orders will be billed at individual rate until proof of status is received. Foreign air speed delivery is included in all Clinics' subscription prices. All prices are subject to change without notice. **POSTMASTER:** Send address changes to *Medical Clinics of North America*, Elsevier Health Sciences Division, Subscription Customer Service, 3251 Riverport Lane, Maryland Heights, MO 63043. **Customer Service: Telephone: 1-800-654-2452** (U.S. and Canada); **1-314-447-8871** (outside U.S. and Canada). **Fax: 314-447-8029. E-mail: journalscustomerserviceusa@ elsevier.com** (for print support); **journalsonlinesupport-usa@elsevier.com** (for online support).

Reprints. For copies of 100 or more of articles in this publication, please contact the Commercial Reprints Department, Elsevier Inc., 360 Park Avenue South, New York, NY 10010-1710. Tel.: 212-633-3874; Fax: 212-633-3820; E-mail: reprints@elsevier.com.

Medical Clinics of North America is also published in Spanish by McGraw-Hill Interamericana Editores S. A., P.O. Box 5-237, 06500 Mexico, D.F., Mexico.

Medical Clinics of North America is covered in *MEDLINE/PubMed (Index Medicus), Current Contents, ASCA, Excerpta Medica, Science Citation Index, and ISI/BIOMED.*

PROGRAM OBJECTIVE

The goal of the *Medical Clinics of North America* is to keep practicing physicians up to date with current clinical practice by providing timely articles reviewing the state of the art in patient care.

TARGET AUDIENCE

All practicing physicians and other healthcare professionals.

LEARNING OBJECTIVES

Upon completion of this activity, participants will be able to:

1. Review the importance of preventive medicine and concrete actions clinicians can take to deliver whole health care.
2. Explain the positive outcomes early cancer detection tests have had on newly diagnosed cancers.
3. Discuss the challenges frontline practicing physicians face while implementing the latest guidelines, as they relate to primary care management of chronic pain and opioid use disorder.

ACCREDITATION

The Elsevier Office of Continuing Medical Education (EOCME) is accredited by the Accreditation Council for Continuing Medical Education (ACCME) to provide continuing medical education for physicians.

The EOCME designates this journal-based CME activity for a maximum of 14 *AMA PRA Category 1 Credit*(s)™. Physicians should claim only the credit commensurate with the extent of their participation in the activity.

All other healthcare professionals requesting continuing education credit for this enduring material will be issued a certificate of participation.

DISCLOSURE OF CONFLICTS OF INTEREST

The EOCME assesses conflict of interest with its instructors, faculty, planners, and other individuals who are in a position to control the content of CME activities. All relevant conflicts of interest that are identified are thoroughly vetted by EOCME for fair balance, scientific objectivity, and patient care recommendations. EOCME is committed to providing its learners with CME activities that promote improvements or quality in healthcare and not a specific proprietary business or a commercial interest.

The planning committee, staff, authors, and editors listed below have identified no financial relationships or relationships to products or devices they or their spouse/life partner have with commercial interest related to the content of this CME activity:
Sara Al-Dahir, PharmD, PhD; Benjamin Buchholz, MPH; William Carroll, MD, Steven Cole, MD, MA; D. Tyler Coyle, MD, MS, Alecia Cyprian, PhD; Joshua L. Denson, MD, MSCR; Deirdra Frum-Vassallo, PhD; Darie Gilliam, DNP; Stephenie Harris; Linda Hill, MD, MPH; Peter J. Hotez, MD, PhD; Shawna Hudson, PhD; Yuri Jadotte, MD, PhD, MPH; Peter T. Katzmarzyk, PhD; Alex H. Krist, MD, MPH; Marie Krousel-Wood, MD, MSPH; Harold Kudler, MD; Dorothy S. Lane, MD, MPH; Michelle Littlejohn; Thomas Locke, MD, MPH; Janelle MacPherson; Marc Meisnere, MHS; Ryan Moran, MD, MPH; Diem Nguyen; Merlin Packiam; Katie Parnellf; Erin Peacock, PhD, MPH; Elizabeth Salisbury-Afshar, MD, MPH; Leia Y. Saltzman, PhD, MSW; Sara J. Singer, PhD, MBA; Kabrina Smith; Robert A. Smith, PhD; Jeannette E. South-Paul, MD, DHL(Hon); Ron Stout, MD, MPH; Jill Waalen, MD, MS, MPH; Shondra Williams, PhD; LaKeisha Williams, PharmD, MSPH; Gary Wiltz, MD; Keith Winfrey, MD, MPH; Catherine Takacs Witkop, MD, PhD, MPH

The planning committee, staff, authors, and editors listed below have identified financial relationships or relationships to products or devices they or their spouse/life partner have with commercial interest related to the content of this CME activity:
Wayne Dysinger, MD, MPH: Employment: Lifestyle Medical

Michael D. Parkinson, MD, MPH, FACPM: Employment: P3 Health Partners

UNAPPROVED/OFF-LABEL USE DISCLOSURE

The EOCME requires CME faculty to disclose to the participants;

1. When products or procedures being discussed are off-label, unlabelled, experimental, and/or investigational (not US Food and Drug Administration [FDA] approved); and
2. Any limitations on the information presented, such as data that are preliminary or that represent ongoing research, interim analyses, and/or unsupported opinions. Faculty may discuss information about pharmaceutical agents that is outside of FDA-approved labelling. This information is intended solely for CME and is not intended to promote off-label use of these medications. If you have any questions, contact the medical affairs department of the manufacturer for the most recent prescribing information.

TO ENROLL

To enroll in the *Medical Clinics of North America* Continuing Medical Education program, call customer service at 1-800-654-2452 or sign up online at http://www.theclinics.com/home/cme. The CME program is available to subscribers for an additional annual fee of USD $319.00.

METHOD OF PARTICIPATION

In order to claim credit, participants must complete the following;
1. Complete enrolment as indicated above.
2. Read the activity.
3. Complete the CME Test and Evaluation. Participants must achieve a score of 70% on the test. All CME Tests and Evaluations must be completed online.

CME INQUIRIES/SPECIAL NEEDS

For all CME inquiries or special needs, please contact elsevierCME@elsevier.com.

MEDICAL CLINICS OF NORTH AMERICA

Contributors

CONSULTING EDITOR

JACK ENDE, MD, MACP
The Schaeffer Professor of Medicine, Perelman School of Medicine of the University of Pennsylvania, Philadelphia, Pennsylvania

EDITOR

MARIE KROUSEL-WOOD, MD, MSPH, FACPM, FAHA
Professor of Medicine and The Jack Aron Chair in Primary Care Medicine; Professor of Epidemiology; Director, Tulane Center for Health Outcomes, Implementation, and Community-Engaged Science (CHOICES); Associate Provost for the Health Sciences; Senior Associate Dean for Faculty Affairs in Medicine; Associate Dean for Public Health and Medical Education; Tulane University School of Medicine and School of Public Health and Tropical Medicine, New Orleans, Louisiana

AUTHORS

SARA AL-DAHIR, PHARMD, PhD
Clinical Professor, Division of Clinical and Administrative Sciences, Xavier University of Louisiana College of Pharmacy, New Orleans, Louisiana

BENJAMIN BUCHHOLZ, MPH
Sickle Cell Center of Excellence, College of Medicine, Howard University, Washington, DC

WILLIAM CARROLL, MD
Department of Medicine, David Geffen School of Medicine, University of California, Los Angeles, California

STEVEN COLE, MD, MA
Professor, Department of Psychiatry, Renaissance School of Medicine, Stony Brook University, Stony Brook, New York; Departments of Scientific Education and Psychiatry, Zucker SOM at Hofstra/Northwell, Hempstead, New York

DAVID TYLER COYLE, MD, MS
Assistant Professor, University of Colorado School of Medicine, Aurora, Colorado

ALECIA CYPRIAN, PhD
Chief Executive Officer, Southeast Community Health Systems, Zachary, Louisiana

JOSHUA L. DENSON, MD
Assistant Professor, Department of Medicine, Tulane University School of Medicine, New Orleans, Louisiana

WAYNE DYSINGER, MD, MPH
Chief Executive Officer, Lifestyle Medical, Riverside, California

DEIRDRA FRUM-VASSALLO, PhD
Health Promotion Disease Prevention, Northport VA Medical Center, Northport, New York

DARIE GILLIAM, DNP
RKM Primary Care, Clinton, Louisiana

STEPHENIE HARRIS
Chief Operations Officer, CommuniHealth Services, Bastrop, Louisiana

LINDA HILL, MD, MPH
Distinguished Professor, Herbert Wertheim School of Public Health, University of California San Diego, La Jolla, California

PETER J. HOTEZ, MD, PhD
Professor, Department of Pediatrics and Molecular Virology and Microbiology, Texas Children's Hospital Center for Vaccine Development, National School of Tropical Medicine, Baylor College of Medicine, Texas Medical Center, Houston, Texas

SHAWNA V. HUDSON, PhD
Professor, Department of Family Medicine and Community Health, Robert Wood Johnson Medical School, New Brunswick, New Jersey

YURI JADOTTE, MD, PhD, MPH
Assistant Professor, Department of Family, Population, and Preventive Medicine, Renaissance School of Medicine, Stony Brook University, Stony Brook, New York; Northeast Institute for Evidence Synthesis and Translation, Division of Nursing Science, School of Nursing, Rutgers University, Newark New Jersey

PETER T. KATZMARZYK, PhD
Professor, Pennington Biomedical Research Center, Baton Rouge, Louisiana

ALEX H. KRIST, MD, MPH
Associate professor, Department of Family Medicine and Population Health, Virginia Commonwealth University, Richmond, Virginia; Inova Fairfax Family Practice Residency, Fairfax, Virginia

MARIE KROUSEL-WOOD, MD, MSPH, FACPM, FAHA
Professor of Medicine and The Jack Aron Chair in Primary Care Medicine; Professor of Epidemiology; Director, Tulane Center for Health Outcomes, Implementation, and Community-Engaged Science (CHOICES); Associate Provost for the Health Sciences; Senior Associate Dean for Faculty Affairs in Medicine; Associate Dean for Public Health and Medical Education; Tulane University School of Medicine and School of Public Health and Tropical Medicine, New Orleans, Louisiana

HAROLD KUDLER, MD
Associate Consulting Professor, Department of Psychiatry and Behavioral Sciences, Duke University, Department of Psychiatry, Uniformed Services University of the Health Sciences, Durham, North Carolina

DOROTHY S. LANE, MD, MPH
SUNY Distinguished Service Professor, Vice Chair, Department of Family, Population and Preventive Medicine, Associate Dean for CME, Renaissance School of Medicine, Stony Brook University, Stony Brook, New York

THOMAS LOCKE, MD, MPH
Resident Physician, University of Colorado School of Medicine, Aurora, Colorado

JANELLE MacPHERSON
BAP Professional Network, Longboat Key, FL

MARC MEISNERE, MHS
National Academies of Sciences, Engineering, and Medicine, Bethesda, Maryland

RYAN MORAN, MD, MPH
Associate Clinical Professor, Department of Medicine, School of Medicine, University of California San Diego, La Jolla, California

DIEM NGUYEN, PHARMD
Chief Executive Officer, NOELA Community Health Center, New Orleans, Louisiana

MICHAEL D. PARKINSON, MD, MPH, FACPM
Principal, P3 Health, LLC (Prevention, Performance, Productivity), Pittsburgh, Pennsylvania

KATIE PARNELL
Chief Executive Officer, CommuniHealth Services, Bastrop, Louisiana

ERIN PEACOCK, PhD, MPH
Assistant Professor, Department of Medicine, Tulane University School of Medicine, Center for Health Outcomes, Implementation, and Community-Engaged Science (CHOICES), Tulane University School of Medicine, New Orleans, Louisiana

ELIZABETH SALISBURY-AFSHAR, MD, MPH
Associate Professor, University of Wisconsin School of Medicine and Public Health, Madison, Wisconsin

LEIA Y. SALTZMAN, PhD, MSW
Assistant Professor, Tulane University School of Social Work, New Orleans, Louisiana

SARA J. SINGER, PhD, MBA
Professor, Department of Medicine, Stanford University School of Medicine, Stanford, California

KABRINA SMITH
Chief Operations Officer, CareSouth Medical and Dental, Baton Rouge, Louisiana

ROBERT A. SMITH, PhD
Senior Vice-President, Early Cancer Detection Science Department, American Cancer Society, Atlanta, Georgia

JEANNETTE E. SOUTH PAUL, MD, DHL(HON)
Office of the Provost, Meharry Medical College, Nashville, Tennessee

RON STOUT, MD, MPH
President and CEO, Ardmore Institute of Health, Ardmore, Oklahoma

JILL WAALEN, MD, MS, MPH
Director-Elect and Adjunct Associate Professor, University of California, San Diego/San Diego State University, General Preventive Medicine Residency Program & Scripps Research Translational Institute, La Jolla, California

LAKEISHA WILLIAMS, PHARMD, MSPH
Clinical Associate Professor, Division of Clinical and Administrative Sciences, Xavier University of Louisiana College of Pharmacy, Center for Minority Health and Health Disparities Research and Education, Xavier University of Louisiana College of Pharmacy, New Orleans, Louisiana

SHONDRA WILLIAMS, PhD
Chief Executive Officer, InclusivCare, Avondale, Louisiana

MICHELLE WILSON, MPH
Program Manager, Department of Medicine, Tulane University School of Medicine, Center for Health Outcomes, Implementation, and Community-Engaged Science (CHOICES), Tulane University School of Medicine, New Orleans, Louisiana

GARY WILTZ, MD
Chief Executive Officer, Teche Action Clinic, Franklin, Louisiana

KEITH WINFREY, MD, MPH
Chief Medical Officer, NOELA Community Health Center, New Orleans, Louisiana

CATHERINE TAKACS WITKOP, MD, PhD, MPH
Professor of Preventive Medicine and Gynecologic Surgery & Obstetrics, Uniformed Services University of the Health Sciences, Bethesda, Maryland

Contents

Throughout the coronavirus disease 2019 (COVID-19) pandemic, there have been numerous demands on primary care practices and providers affecting work engagement and burnout, which can affect health-care delivery and patient outcomes. We determined potentially modifiable factors associated with work engagement among employees of federally qualified health centers (FQHCs) throughout Louisiana. Resilient coping, spirituality, and social support were associated with being engaged at work. FQHC employees perceiving a more chaotic work environment and those with depressive or anxiety symptoms were less likely to be engaged at work. Being engaged was associated with confidence in COVID-19 vaccine recommendation for adults.

Global immunization programs have saved tens of millions of lives over the last 2 decades. Now, the recent successes of COVID-19 vaccines having saved more than 3 million lives in North America during the pandemic may open the door to accelerate technologies for other emerging infection vaccines. New vaccines for respiratory syncytial virus, norovirus, influenza, herpes simplex virus, shingles, dengue fever, enteric bacterial infections, malaria, and Chagas disease are advancing through clinical development and could become ready for delivery over the next 5 years. The successful delivery of these new vaccines may require expanded advocacy and communications efforts.

Although cancer has been the second leading cause of death for close to 100 years, progress has been made in reducing cancer mortality and morbidity, with the adoption of high-quality screening tests and treatment advances delivered at earlier stages of diagnosis. To achieve the high cancer screening rates demonstrated by some practices, proven effective strategies need to be broadly adopted at both the patient and population levels. Factors affecting cancer screening test completion and approaches to improvement are described both generally and for breast, lung, cervical, colorectal, and prostate cancers. Closing the racial disparity gap is a critical component of reaching cancer screening and prevention goals.

Clinicians play an important role in the prevention of unintentional injuries. Falls and motor vehicle crashes (MVC) have predictable and overlapping antecedents. Systematic screening for and management of vision impairment, frailty, cognitive impairment, polypharmacy, and inappropriate medications will reduce both falls and MVC risks. Fall-prevention measures, such as strength training, need to be more widely prescribed by physicians and implemented by older adults. Technologically tailored approaches are needed to leverage fall-reduction programs at home, as well as education of older adults regarding home hazards.

Evidence-based clinical preventive services have the potential to reduce morbidity and mortality and optimize health. The Affordable Care Act mandates coverage without cost-sharing for several clinical preventive services. The Women's Preventive Services Initiative (WPSI) has worked to and continues to identify gaps in recommended preventive services for women. The WPSI Well-Woman Chart and the accompanying Clinical Summary Tables can be used at the point of care to ensure women are offered and receive all the preventive services recommended for their age and circumstance.

The prevalence of obesity continues to increase in the United States and globally, placing a large portion of the population at an increased risk of metabolic and cardiovascular diseases. Primary care settings remain the main access point for medical care and preventive medical services for most individuals and thus represent a key environment for treating and managing obesity. Several recent pragmatic trials conducted in primary care have demonstrated clinically significant weight loss and associated reductions in chronic disease risk factors, highlighting the need to translate these programs into mainstream clinical care.

The medical community has proposed several clinical recommendations to promote patient safety and health amid the opioid overdose public health crisis. For a frontline practicing physician, distilling the evidence and implementing the latest guidelines may prove challenging. This article aims to highlight pertinent updates and clinical care pearls as they relate to primary care management of chronic pain and opioid use disorder.

systems, including the Veterans Health Administration and the nation, to scale and spread a whole health approach to care. The report identifies 5 foundational elements for whole health care and sets 6 national, state, and local policy goals for change. This article summarizes the report, emphasizes the importance of preventive medicine, and identifies concrete actions clinicians and practices can take now to deliver whole health care.

Foreword

Providing Preventive Services: Challenges We Can and Must Meet

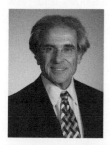

Jack Ende, MD, MACP
Consulting Editor

For the busy clinician, providing patients with appropriate preventive services is not without its challenges. Here I identify three: knowledge, systems, and will. Each is important, but perhaps "will" challenges us most.

The first challenge is the "what" that is, what preventive services are associated with the best outcomes for the patient in front of you? Should this 62-year-old man without a family history of colorectal cancer be screened with colonoscopy, or is some other less-invasive test sufficient? And if it is, how often should it be performed? This is an example of the knowledge base of preventive medicine that all practicing clinicians should have at hand. Fortunately, with today's point-of-care information systems, that knowledge is readily available. So, this first challenge associated with providing preventive services is not so hard.

The second challenge is actually delivering the service, ie, getting the patient to agree with the recommended preventive service, gaining access to the service, and getting it paid for. This often brings into focus the unfortunate inequities of care that characterize our health care system, largely driven by socioeconomic factors, and which has led to the sad observation by many that when it comes to health outcomes, "your zip code may be more important than your genetic code." This challenge is not to be minimized, but there are now several strategies being implemented (some of the best are described in this issue) and, it is hoped, these inequities will yield to policy measures. So, for this challenge, there is hope.

But the final challenge, which I referred to earlier as being determined by "will," is the one that troubles me the most. Here I refer not to knowledge of evidence-based preventive services, and not to the resources in support of the same, but to attitude. Will the busy clinician devote time to counseling for preventive services? Will she or he remember to—or chose to—ask about exposure to firearms, vaccinations, seatbelts,

Med Clin N Am 107 (2023) xv–xvi
https://doi.org/10.1016/j.mcna.2023.07.003
0025-7125/23/© 2023 Published by Elsevier Inc.

domestic violence, loneliness, diet, exercise, and so forth? The list is long; the time we have with patients is short. This challenge is, well, quite challenging.

To a great extent this last challenge can and should be addressed by innovative interventions in care systems (again, several of which are described in this issue) and by modifications in quality measures and, with that, reimbursement. But we should not forget the central role of the clinician, that is, his or her motivation and will to provide all patients with the best possible preventive services.

This issue of *Medical Clinics of North America*, "Current Challenges and New Directions in Preventive Medicine," is informative, empowering, and, I believe, inspirational. It should help move us to meet the challenges associated with providing our patients with the preventive services they need and deserve.

Jack Ende, MD, MACP
Perelman School of Medicine of
the University of Pennsylvania
Philadelphia, PA 19104, USA

E-mail address:
jack.ende@pennmedicine.upenn.edu

Preface

Preventing Disease and Promoting Health: An Update for Clinicians

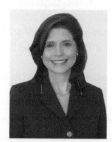

Marie Krousel-Wood, MD, MSPH, FACPM, FAHA
Editor

Prevention is a powerful tool for building health resilience! Prior to the discovery of efficacious medications, medical devices, and procedures, primary prevention of disease defined medical care in North America and beyond. Advances in modern medicine and preventive services delivery have greatly expanded medical care and, more importantly, life expectancy over time. The Accreditation Council for Graduate Medical Education–accredited specialty of preventive medicine was established in 1946, training physicians across the prevention spectrum (primary to tertiary prevention) to practice at the intersection of clinical medicine and public health and improve health for their patients and populations. In addition, the US Preventive Medicine Task Force was created in 1984 as an independent, volunteer panel of national experts in prevention and evidence-based medicine and provides data-driven recommendations about clinical preventive services, such as screenings, counseling services, and preventive medications. Given the importance of prevention among people from prebirth to old age in not only reducing premature morbidity and mortality but also improving health and wellness, the practice of prevention is broadly embraced by preventive medicine physicians, primary care providers, and those in other specialties/subspecialties. The relevance of prevention, public health, and community-engagement was amplified during the COVID-19 pandemic, signaling a critical need for all health care providers and health systems to support healthy communities by implementing evidence-based prevention practices in primary (eg, vaccination), secondary (eg, screening for chronic disease), and tertiary (eg, treatment of existing disease) prevention with specific attention to health equity *before, during, and after* a crisis. Though millions of lives were saved during the pandemic through vaccination and basic prevention measures, widespread uncertainties emerged about the value of primary prevention, leading to suboptimal uptake of preventive services, including vaccination. This reinforced the critical

Med Clin N Am 107 (2023) xvii–xviii
https://doi.org/10.1016/j.mcna.2023.07.002
0025-7125/23/© 2023 Published by Elsevier Inc.

responsibility of physicians and other health care providers in understanding and implementing the evidence and effectively communicating with their patients and communities about risks and benefits. The importance of health care providers as the "most trusted source of health information" was highlighted, and innovative, prevention-based clinical practice models supporting better health outcomes, health resilience, and health equity emerged. There is currently increased attention on public and population health coupled with a call to action to realign our investments in our overall health care infrastructure that support community-engagement with implementation of evidence-based prevention strategies as well as support our clinical and public health workforce—all signaling the enormous potential for transformative health care organizations to change their approach to improving health by focusing on healthy behaviors, prevention, and wellness.

The goal of this issue is to provide clinicians with valuable insights about optimizing uptake and delivery of preventive services to improve health and wellness in the patients and the communities we serve. This collection of articles reviews current challenges and future directions for the practice of preventive medicine within real-world clinical practice. In the first segment, articles focus on primary prevention, including the association between engaged health care workers and confidence in recommending vaccination; the importance of vaccination and the impact of vaccine hesitancy on population health; and challenges for future vaccines implementation. The second segment highlights secondary prevention strategies, including screening for cancer, unintentional injury risk in older adults, alcohol misuse as well as implementing women's preventive services. The third segment features opportunities and new strategies for tertiary prevention, including use of a validated, practical, open access scale for monitoring antihypertensive medication adherence; proven approaches for addressing obesity, pain management, and opioid use disorder; and existing/emerging tools for counseling patients and integrating mHealth in clinical practice. The final, culminating segment presents novel and evolving prevention-focused practice models—"Lifestyle Medicine" and "Whole Health Systems" (the latter builds on a recent report by the National Academy of Sciences, Engineering and Medicine)—aimed at engaging individuals, their communities, and health systems in preventing disease and promoting health for all.

In summary, this issue provides evidence-based updates by experts in the fields of preventive medicine and primary care and includes clinical and public health practice recommendations and tools for screening and treatment. In addition, future directions with innovative health models for implementing primary, secondary, and tertiary preventive medicine services are described. The articles highlight the power of prevention in building *health resilience, optimizing health outcomes, and advancing health equity* for our patients and communities.

Marie Krousel-Wood, MD, MSPH, FACPM, FAHA
Tulane University School of Medicine and Tulane University
School of Public Health and Tropical Medicine
Tulane Center for Health Outcomes, implementation
and Community-Engaged Science (CHOICES)
1430 Tulane Avenue
New Orleans, LA 70112, USA

E-mail address:
mawood@tulane.edu

Health-care Worker Engagement in Federally Qualified Health Centers and Associations with Confidence in Making Health-care Recommendations

Evidence from the Louisiana Community Engagement Alliance

Erin Peacock, PhD, MPH[a,b,]*, Leia Y. Saltzman, PhD, MSW[c],
Joshua L. Denson, MD, MSCR[a], Sara Al-Dahir, PharmD, PhD[d],
Michelle Wilson, MPH[a,b], Alecia Cyprian, PhD[e], Darie Gilliam, DNP[f],
Stephenie Harris[g], Katie Parnell[g], Diem Nguyen, PharmD[h],
Kabrina Smith, MS, MPH[i], Shondra Williams, PhD[j], Gary Wiltz, MD[k],
Keith Winfrey, MD, MPH[h], LaKeisha Williams, PharmD, MSPH[d,l],
Marie Krousel-Wood, MD, MSPH[a,b,m]

Sources of Funding: Research reported in this NIH Community Engagement Alliance (CEAL) Against COVID-19 Disparities publication was supported by the National Institutes of Health under Award Number OT2 HL158260. The authors also receive NIH funding from R01 HL133790 (Krousel-Wood – Multi PI, Peacock – Study Manager), R01 HL153750 (Krousel-Wood – PI; Peacock – Co-Investigator), R33 AG068481 (Krousel-Wood & Peacock – Co-Investigators), K12 HD043451 (Krousel-Wood – PI; Peacock – Data Analyst), U54 GM104940 (Krousel-Wood), U54 TR001368 (Krousel-Wood), and 5U54MD007595-14 (Williams). The content is solely the responsibility of the authors and does not necessarily represent the official views of the National Institutes of Health.

[a] Department of Medicine, Tulane University School of Medicine, 1430 Tulane Avenue, New Orleans, LA 70112, USA; [b] Center for Health Outcomes, Implementation, and Community-Engaged Science (CHOICES), Tulane University School of Medicine, 1430 Tulane Avenue, New Orleans, LA 70112, USA; [c] Tulane University School of Social Work, 127 Elk Place, New Orleans, LA 70112, USA; [d] Division of Clinical and Administrative Sciences, Xavier University of Louisiana College of Pharmacy, 1 Drexel Drive, New Orleans, LA 70125, USA; [e] Southeast Community Health Systems, 6351 Main Street, Zachary, LA 70791, USA; [f] RKM Primary Care, 11990 Jackson Street, Clinton, LA 70722, USA; [g] CommuniHealth Services, 314 N Franklin Street, Bastrop, LA 71220, USA; [h] NOELA Community Health Center, 13805 Chef Menteur Highway, New Orleans, LA 70129, USA; [i] CareSouth Medical and Dental, 3111 Florida Street, Baton Rouge, LA 70806, USA; [j] InclusivCare, 4028 US Highway 90, Avondale, LA 70094, USA; [k] Teche Action Clinic, 1115 Weber Street, Franklin, LA 70538, USA; [l] Center for Minority Health and Health Disparities Research and Education, Xavier University of Louisiana College of Pharmacy, 1 Drexel Drive, New Orleans, LA 70125, USA; [m] Department of Epidemiology, Tulane University School of Public Health and Tropical Medicine, 1440 Canal Street, New Orleans, LA 70112, USA
* Corresponding author. Department of Medicine, Tulane University School of Medicine, 1440 Canal Street, Suite 1604, New Orleans, LA 70112.
E-mail address: epeacoc@tulane.edu

Med Clin N Am 107 (2023) 963–977
https://doi.org/10.1016/j.mcna.2023.06.009
0025-7125/23/© 2023 Elsevier Inc. All rights reserved.

KEYWORDS

- COVID-19 • Trusted messenger • Vaccine/booster uptake
- Health-care worker burnout/engagement • Race differences

KEY POINTS

- Throughout the COVID-19 pandemic, there have been numerous demands on health-care workers, leading to impacts on work engagement and burnout, which can affect health-care delivery and patient outcomes.
- This study aimed to identify potentially modifiable factors associated with work engagement (ie, *lack* of burnout) among health-care workers in federally qualified health centers. In this sample, resilient coping, spirituality, and social support were associated with being engaged at work.
- Employees with symptoms of depression or anxiety and those perceiving a more chaotic work environment were less likely to be engaged at work.
- The associations between symptoms of depression/anxiety and lower odds of being engaged, and between high social support and higher odds of being engaged, were stronger for those in patient care roles versus nonpatient care roles, whereas high resilient coping had a stronger association with work engagement for those in nonpatient care versus patient care roles.
- Work engagement was associated with being confident in recommending adult COVID-19 vaccination.

INTRODUCTION

In early 2020, high coronavirus disease 2019 (COVID-19)-associated morbidity and mortality coupled with alarming health disparities, the changing COVID-19 landscape and guidelines, widespread uncertainty, and mis/disinformation about COVID-19 preventive strategies[1] prompted an urgent need for community-engaged strategies to disseminate accurate, relevant, and timely information about COVID-19. The Community Engagement Alliance (CEAL) was funded by the National Institutes of Health to rapidly engage communities hardest-hit by the COVID-19 pandemic and provide trustworthy, science-based information through active community engagement and outreach.[2] Identified early on as a "COVID-19 hotspot" area, Louisiana was one of the initial CEAL awardees and was able to engage quickly through established alliances with federally qualified health centers (FQHCs) and other state-wide community partners. Early Louisiana CEAL (LA-CEAL) efforts focused on identifying and equipping "trusted messengers" to deliver accurate and timely information to support people's decision-making about COVID-19 vaccination and other preventive strategies.

Widespread trust in health-care workers as a source of COVID-19 information is well documented[3–5]; yet less is known about the factors associated with health-care workers' COVID-19-related actions, attitudes, and recommendations. FQHCs are health centers that provide comprehensive primary care and preventive health services in a designated medically underserved area or to a medically underserved population.[6] Similar to other front-line segments of the health-care sector, FQHCs have encountered multiple challenges during the COVID-19 era, including keeping apace of changing COVID-19 information and guidelines; pivoting resources from other preventive and chronic disease care to COVID-19 testing, vaccination, and treatment;

staff shortages due to COVID-19-related absence; and high staff turnover.[7] In addition, health-care workers at FQHCs experience additional stress associated with serving a patient population with poor health outcomes and high exposure to detrimental social determinants of health.[8]

Since the onset of the COVID-19 pandemic, there has been increasing concern regarding health-care worker burnout across health systems and its impact on health system functioning and achievement of positive patient outcomes.[9,10] Using a positive deviance approach that seeks to understand why some individuals do *not* experience the same negative outcomes experienced by their peers,[11] the purpose of this study was to determine modifiable factors associated with work engagement (ie, *lack* of burnout) among employees (patient care and nonpatient care) of LA-CEAL's partner FQHCs in Louisiana. Furthermore, associations between being engaged at work and health-care worker actions (COVID-19 booster uptake) and attitudes (self-efficacy in delivering COVID-19 vaccination information; confidence in strongly recommending adult vaccination) were explored. Differences between those in patient care versus nonpatient care roles were explored for insights to inform the development of interventions to improve work engagement among health-care workers. Due to hypothesized race differences in burnout,[12,13] differences across Black respondents and those who were not Black were explored.

METHODS
Study Population and Data Collection

A cross-sectional survey was conducted among 472 employees of clinics from 8 partner FQHCs throughout Louisiana between October and December 2022. In collaboration with the FQHC leadership, all FQHC employees (both patient care and nonpatient care) were invited to participate via an email from the LA-CEAL research team. Questionnaires were self-administered via REDCap following the validation of an organizational email address. The study was approved by the Tulane University Institutional Review Board. All human subjects procedures were in accordance with institutional guidelines. Participants provided informed consent and were compensated for participation.

Study Measures

Engagement at work
We used the 22-item validated Maslach Burnout Inventory (MBI) for Medical Personnel,[14,a] measuring feelings across 3 subscales: emotional exhaustion (Cronbach's alpha = 0.93 in this sample), depersonalization (Cronbach's alpha = 0.64), and personal accomplishment (Cronbach's alpha = 0.85). For each subscale, mean scores across subscale items were calculated and then dichotomized into high versus low using critical boundaries based on population norms.[15] Participants were categorized into burnout profiles based on high versus low ratings across each subscale.

- Engaged = low emotional exhaustion, low depersonalization, high personal accomplishment
- Ineffective = low emotional exhaustion, low depersonalization, low personal accomplishment
- Overextended = high emotional exhaustion, low depersonalization, personal accomplishment not specified

- Disengaged = low emotional exhaustion, high depersonalization, personal accomplishment not specified
- Burnout = high emotional exhaustion, high depersonalization, personal accomplishment not specified

Finally, burnout profiles were dichotomized as "engaged" versus other (ie, ineffective, overextended, disengaged, and burnout).

Potential factors

The survey captured demographics (race, gender, age, residential zip code, work role, years in work role), mental health history, resilient coping, spirituality, social support, and organizational culture. Race was dichotomized as Black versus not Black. Residential zip codes were matched to data in the Federal Office of Rural Health Policy data files[16] to determine rural versus not rural residence. Health-care work role was collected using predefined categories (administrator, dentist, medical assistant, nurse, nurse practitioner, outreach staff, patient support staff, pharmacist, physician, physician assistant, other); all responses, including open-ended "other" responses, were grouped into *patient care* (nonprovider clinical roles, eg, nurses, medical assistants, dental assistants, pharmacy technicians; providers, eg, nurse practitioners, physicians, dentists, pharmacists, and licensed therapists) versus *nonpatient care* roles (administrators and nonclinical personnel, eg, front desk, billing). Symptoms of depression and anxiety were measured using the 2-item Patient Health Questionnaire[17] and 2-item Generalized Anxiety Disorder,[18] respectively. Resilient coping was measured using the 4-item Brief Resilient Coping Scale[19] and categorized per published scoring criteria into low/medium versus high resilient coping. Spirituality was measured using 6 items chosen from the 22-item Spirituality Scale[20]; participants falling in the highest tertile of the distribution of mean scores across items were categorized as having high spirituality. Social support was measured using the 12-item Multidimensional Scale of Perceived Social Support[21] and categorized into low/moderate versus high social support using published scoring guidelines. Organizational culture was measured using the 22-item Practice Culture Assessment[22] across 3 domains: Change Culture (collaboration on quality improvement and problem resolution), Work Culture (positive and productive work environment), and Chaos (instability and disruption).

Coronavirus disease 2019-related actions and attitudes

Three outcomes related to health-care workers' COVID-19-related actions/attitudes were measured. *COVID-19 booster uptake* was measured using a single survey item, "Have you received at least one COVID-19 booster shot?" *Self-efficacy* was measured using a 5-point Likert response to de novo questions (presented in **Fig. 1**) about confidence in delivering information about COVID-19 vaccination (eg, engaging people in conversations about why they are hesitant to get vaccinated, answering questions about child vaccination) (Cronbach's alpha in this sample = 0.93). A mean score across all 8 items was computed and high self-efficacy was defined as the highest tertile of the distribution of summary scores. Finally, *confidence in recommending the vaccine in adults* was defined as a response of "somewhat" or "very" confident to the question, "How confident are you in strongly recommending to an adult that they get vaccinated against COVID-19?"

Statistical Analysis

Participant characteristics were summarized using proportions or means and standard deviations as appropriate. Design-corrected Pearson's chi-squared and simple

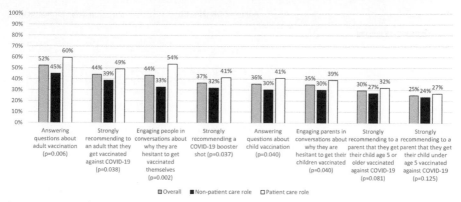

Fig. 1. Percent of respondents at least somewhat confident in delivering COVID-19 vaccination information (n = 472) *P*-value from design-corrected Pearson's chi-squared test comparing those in nonpatient care versus patient care role.

linear regression models with robust standard errors to account for clustering at the FQHC level were used to test for differences in participant characteristics and MBI profile across role (nonpatient care versus patient care) and race (Black versus not Black). Multivariable logistic regression with robust standard errors was used to estimate adjusted odds ratios (aOR) and 95% confidence intervals (CIs) for being engaged at work. Health-care worker role-stratified and race-stratified models, respectively, were used to identify potential differences between participants in non-patient care roles versus patient care roles, and Black participants versus those who were not Black. Separate multivariable logistic regression models with robust standard errors explored the association between being engaged at work and the 3 COVID-19-related actions/attitudes, overall and stratified by health care worker role (nonpatient care versus patient care) and race (Black versus not Black). Effect modification by health-care worker role and race was tested by including an *engaged x role* or *engaged x race* interaction term in overall models and role-stratified and race-stratified results were presented. All analyses were done using Stata 14.2 (StataCorp, College Station, TX). **Fig. 2** was created using R 3.4.3 (R Foundation for Statistical Computing, Vienna, Austria).

RESULTS
Participant Characteristics

Participant characteristics are presented in **Table 1**. The sample was 54.2% Black, 94.7% women, and 33.8% rural, with a mean age of 42.8 years (SD 11.8). The "not Black" sample was made up of 196 participants identifying as White, 4 participants identifying as Asian, 1 participant identifying as American Indian/Alaska Native, and 5 participants identifying as having more than one race. Patient care employees made up 51.1% of the sample, including nonprovider clinical roles (33.1%) and providers (17.9%), with the other 48.9% in nonpatient care roles (administrators [7.5%] and nonclinical personnel [41.5%]). On average, participants had been working in their role for 10.1 years (SD 9.2) and 19.1% indicated experiencing symptoms consistent with depression or anxiety.

Participants in patient care roles were more likely than those not in patient care roles to have high spirituality (33.5% vs 25.8%, *P* = .031), to be engaged at work (43.1% vs 31.0%, *P* = .005), to have high self-efficacy in delivering COVID-19 vaccination

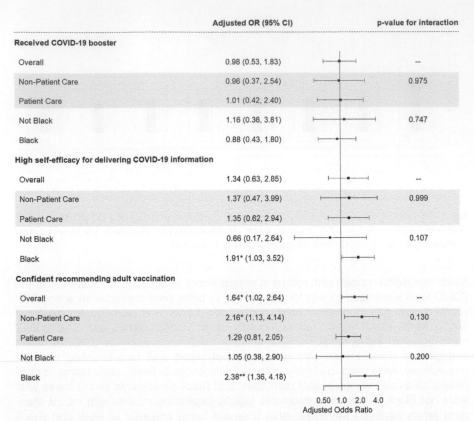

	Adjusted OR (95% CI)		p-value for interaction
Received COVID-19 booster			
Overall	0.98 (0.53, 1.83)		--
Non-Patient Care	0.96 (0.37, 2.54)		0.975
Patient Care	1.01 (0.42, 2.40)		
Not Black	1.16 (0.36, 3.81)		0.747
Black	0.88 (0.43, 1.80)		
High self-efficacy for delivering COVID-19 information			
Overall	1.34 (0.63, 2.85)		--
Non-Patient Care	1.37 (0.47, 3.99)		0.999
Patient Care	1.35 (0.62, 2.94)		
Not Black	0.66 (0.17, 2.64)		0.107
Black	1.91* (1.03, 3.52)		
Confident recommending adult vaccination			
Overall	1.64* (1.02, 2.64)		--
Non-Patient Care	2.16* (1.13, 4.14)		0.130
Patient Care	1.29 (0.81, 2.05)		
Not Black	1.05 (0.38, 2.90)		0.200
Black	2.38** (1.36, 4.18)		

0.50 1.0   2.0   4.0
Adjusted Odds Ratio

Fig. 2. Overall and subgroup associations between work engagement and COVID-19-related actions and attitudes among health-care workers in FQHCs. OR, odds ratio; CI, confidence interval; [a] $P < .001$, [b] $P < .01$, [c] $P < .05$. All models adjusted for race, gender, age, rural residence, patient care role, time in role, symptoms of depression or anxiety minus the stratifying variable. p-interactions from overall models with *engaged x patient care* or *engaged x race* interaction term.

information (36.8% vs 25.3%, $P = .011$), and to be confident in recommending adult vaccination (49.2% vs 38.9%, $P = .038$). Compared with those in nonpatient care roles, those in patient care roles also had served longer in their roles on average (11.5 years [SD 9.9] vs 8.7 years [SD 8.3], $P = .043$) and had lower average Change Culture and Work Culture scores (Change Culture: 63.5 [SD 22.3] vs 70.4 [SD 22.2], $P = .010$; Work Culture: 62.0 [SD 21.0] vs 66.2 [SD 21.3], $P = .009$). Black participants were more likely than participants who were not Black to have high resilient coping (45.2% vs 27.8%, respectively; $P = .004$), to have received a COVID-19 booster shot (56.2% vs 36.8%, respectively; $P = .009$), to report high self-efficacy in delivering COVID-19 vaccination information (40.2% vs 19.9%, respectively; $P = .015$), and to report confidence in strongly recommending adult vaccination against COVID-19 (51.6% vs 35.9% confident, respectively; $P = .007$).

Work Engagement

The mean scores for the 3 MBI subscales were 1.54 (SD 1.40) for emotional exhaustion, 0.66 (SD 0.91) for depersonalization, and 4.12 (SD 1.45) for personal

Table 1
Participant characteristics, LA-CEAL Trusted Messenger survey, October-December 2022

	Overall (n = 472)	By Health-care Worker Role			By Race		
		Non-patient Care Role (n = 229)	Patient Care Role (n = 239)	p-value	Not Black (n = 206) % (n)	Black (n = 244) % (n)	p-value
Black, % (n)	54.2 (244)	61.8 (134)	46.3 (106)	0.066	—	—	—
Woman, % (n)	94.7 (445)	93.9 (214)	95.4 (228)	0.477	94.2 (194)	95.0 (230)	0.727
Age, Mean (SD)	42.8 (11.8)	43.2 (12.1)	42.4 (11.6)	0.633	42.4 (11.9)	43.1 (11.8)	0.431
Rural, % (n)	33.8 (158)	37.2 (84)	31.2 (74)	0.378	40.8 (84)	29.6 (71)	0.147
Patient care role, % (n)	51.1 (239)	—	—	—	59.7 (123)	44.2 (106)	0.066
Years in work role, Mean (SD)	10.1 (9.2)	8.7 (8.3)	**11.5 (9.9)**	**0.043**	10.0 (9.8)	10.2 (8.8)	0.731
Symptoms of depression/anxiety, % (n)	19.1 (90)	21.4 (49)	17.2 (41)	0.329	22.3 (46)	15.2 (37)	0.056
High resilient coping, % (n)	37.6 (176)	37.6 (85)	37.7 (90)	0.993	**27.8 (57)**	**45.2 (109)**	**0.004**
High spirituality, % (n)	29.5 (139)	**25.8 (59)**	**33.5 (80)**	**0.031**	27.2 (56)	31.6 (77)	0.204
High social support, % (n)	75.9 (358)	72.9 (167)	78.7 (188)	0.130	81.6 (168)	70.5 (172)	0.056
Change culture score, Mean (SD)	66.9 (22.6)	**70.4 (22.2)**	**63.5 (22.3)**	**0.010**	65.2 (21.8)	68.3 (23.5)	0.374
Work culture score, Mean (SD)	64.1 (21.3)	**56.2 (21.3)**	**62.0 (21.0)**	**0.009**	62.9 (19.5)	65.3 (22.6)	0.349
Chaos score, Mean (SD)	39.2 (21.4)	37.9 (21.4)	40.7 (21.4)	0.293	42.0 (20.2)	37.3 (21.6)	0.149
Engaged, % (n)	36.9 (174)	**31.0 (71)**	**43.1 (103)**	**0.005**	36.9 (76)	38.1 (93)	0.756
Received COVID-19 booster, % (n)	47.6 (203)	45.6 (94)	49.8 (108)	0.455	**36.8 (64)**	**56.2 (131)**	**0.009**
High self-efficacy for delivering COVID-19 vaccination information, % (n)	31.1 (147)	**25.3 (58)**	**36.8 (88)**	**0.011**	**19.9 (41)**	**40.2 (98)**	**0.015**
Confidence in recommending vaccine, % (n)	44.2 (208)	**38.9 (89)**	**49.2 (117)**	**0.038**	**35.9 (74)**	**51.6 (126)**	**0.007**

SD, standard deviation; LA-CEAL, Louisiana Community-Engagement Alliance against COVID-19 Disparities.
BOLD, $P < .05$.

accomplishment, translating into 16.3% of the sample with high emotional exhaustion, 4.5% with high depersonalization, and 58.3% with low personal accomplishment. Summarizing across subscales, 36.9% of the sample had an engaged profile versus 46.0% ineffective, 12.7% overextended, 0.9% disengaged, and 3.6% burnout (**Table 2**). Burnout profiles differed across health-care worker role ($P = .030$), with a higher percent of those in patient care roles than nonpatient care roles categorized as engaged (43.1% vs 31.0%) and a lower percent categorized as ineffective (38.5% vs 52.8%).

Factors Associated with Engagement at Work

In the fully adjusted model (**Table 3**), those in patient care roles had higher odds of being engaged than those in nonpatient care roles (aOR = 1.74, 95% CI 1.22, 2.49). Those with high (versus low/medium) resilient coping, high (versus low/medium) spirituality, and high (versus low/moderate) social support had higher odds of being engaged (aOR = 2.87, 95% CI 1.96, 4.22; aOR = 1.60, 95% CI 1.07, 2.40; aOR = 2.35, 95% CI 1.46, 3.78; respectively). Reporting symptoms of depression/anxiety was associated with lower odds of being engaged (aOR = 0.50, 95% CI 0.31, 0.81). Chaos was associated with lower odds of being engaged (aOR = 0.96, 95% CI 0.94, 0.99).

Health-care worker role and race-stratified models are also presented in **Table 3**. Chaos score was negatively associated with work engagement among those in nonpatient care roles (aOR = 0.97, 95% CI 0.94, 0.99) and patient care roles (aOR = 0.96, 95% CI 0.93, 0.99). Additional factors associated with engagement among those in nonpatient care roles were years in work role (aOR = 0.95, 95% CI 0.91, 1.00), high resilient coping (aOR = 6.03, 95% CI 2.59, 14.01), and work culture score (aOR = 1.03, 95% CI 1.00, 1.05), whereas high social support was associated with higher odds of engagement (aOR = 3.16, 95% CI 1.76, 5.68) among those in patient care roles. Being in a patient care role was associated with work engagement among participants who were not Black (aOR = 2.39, 95% CI 1.33, 4.29). High resilient coping and high social support were associated with being engaged in participants who were not Black (Coping: aOR = 2.35, 95% CI 1.35, 4.11; Social support: aOR = 3.31, 95% CI 1.35, 8.14) and Black participants (Coping: aOR = 3.47, 95% CI 2.15, 5.61; Social support: aOR = 1.93, 95% CI 1.14, 3.28). Among Black participants, Chaos score was negatively associated with being engaged (aOR = 0.96, 95% CI 0.93, 0.99).

Association Between Work Engagement and Coronavirus disease 2019-Related Actions and Attitudes

Overall, 47.6% of participants had received a COVID-19 booster and 44.2% were confident in strongly recommending adult COVID-19 vaccination. Percent of participants confident in delivering other COVID-19 vaccination information ranged from 52.4% for answering questions about adult vaccination to 25.2% for strongly recommending to a parent that they get their child aged younger than 5 years vaccinated against COVID-19 (see **Fig. 1**). Confidence was higher among those in patient care roles versus nonpatient care roles for all messages, although the difference did not reach statistical significance for the 2 messages related to recommending pediatric vaccination.

Having an engaged profile was associated with higher odds of being confident in recommending adult vaccination (aOR = 1.64, 95% CI 1.02, 2.64) (see **Fig. 2**). The association was stronger for Black participants (aOR = 2.38, 95% CI 1.36, 4.18) than participants who were not Black (aOR = 1.05, 95% CI 0.38, 2.90) and for those in nonpatient care roles (aOR = 2.16, 95% CI 1.13, 4.14) versus

Table 2
Maslach Burnout Inventory[a] profiles, LA-CEAL Trusted Messenger survey, October to December 2022

Profile	Emotional Exhaustion	Depersonalization	Personal Accomplishment	Overall (n = 472) % (n)	By Health-care Worker Role		By Race	
					Nonpatient Care Role (n = 229) % (n)	Patient Care Role (n = 239) % (n)	Not Black (n = 206) % (n)	Black (n = 244) % (n)
Engaged	Low	Low	High	36.9 (174)	31.0 (71)	43.1 (103)	36.9 (76)	38.1 (93)
Ineffective	Low	Low	Low	46.0 (217)	52.8 (121)	38.5 (92)	42.2 (87)	49.6 (121)
Overextended	High	Low	High or low	12.7 (60)	11.8 (27)	13.8 (33)	16.0 (33)	9.4 (23)
Disengaged	Low	High	High or low	0.9 (4)	1.8 (4)	0 (0)	0.5 (1)	0.8 (2)
Burnout	High	High	High or low	3.6 (17)	2.6 (6)	4.6 (11)	4.4 (9)	2.1 (5)
p-value					0.030		0.095	

LA-CEAL, Louisiana Community-Engagement Alliance against COVID-19 Disparities.
[a] Copyright ©1981, 2016 by Christina Maslach & Susan E. Jackson All rights reserved in all media. Published by Mind Garden, Inc., www.mindgarden.com.

Table 3
Factors associated with work engagement in federally qualified health centers, overall and by health-care worker role and race

	Overall (n = 394) Adjusted OR (95% CI)	By Health-care Worker Role		By Race	
		Nonpatient Care Role (n = 189) Adjusted OR (95% CI)	Patient Care Role (n = 203) Adjusted OR (95% CI)	Not Black (n = 189) Adjusted OR (95% CI)	Black (n = 207) Adjusted OR (95% CI)
Black	0.94 (0.70, 1.26)	1.49 (0.65, 3.43)	0.82 (0.48, 1.39)	—	—
Woman	1.17 (0.56, 2.42)	3.49 (0.34, 35.82)	0.77 (0.33, 1.77)	0.97 (0.31, 3.00)	1.82 (0.70, 4.74)
Age	1.01 (0.98, 1.05)	1.02 (0.99, 1.05)	1.01 (0.96, 1.07)	1.02 (0.96, 1.08)	1.01 (0.99, 1.03)
Rural	1.24 (0.89, 1.71)	1.79 (0.95, 3.35)	1.09 (0.38, 3.14)	1.27 (0.66, 2.45)	1.40 (0.70, 2.81)
Patient care role	**1.74[b] (1.22, 2.49)**	—	—	**2.39[b] (1.33, 4.29)**	1.31 (0.68, 2.51)
Years in work role	0.98 (0.95, 1.02)	**0.95[c] (0.91, 1.00)**	0.99 (0.94, 1.03)	0.99 (0.93, 1.05)	0.97 (0.94, 1.00)
Symptoms of depression/anxiety	**0.50[c] (0.31, 0.81)**	0.93 (0.55, 1.58)	**0.25[c] (0.07, 0.95)**	0.55 (0.28, 1.08)	0.44 (0.15, 1.26)
High resilient coping	**2.87[a] (1.96, 4.22)**	**6.03[b] (2.59, 14.01)**	1.81 (0.84, 3.89)	**2.35[b] (1.35, 4.11)**	**3.47[a] (2.15, 5.61)**
High spirituality	**1.60[c] (1.07, 2.40)**	1.45 (0.60, 3.48)	1.52 (0.70, 3.32)	1.49 (0.48, 4.67)	1.69 (0.81, 3.50)
High social support	**2.35[b] (1.46, 3.78)**	1.88 (0.78, 4.55)	**3.16[b] (1.76, 5.68)**	**3.31[c] (1.35, 8.14)**	**1.93[c] (1.14, 3.28)**
Change culture score	0.99 (0.97, 1.00)	0.99 (0.98, 1.01)	0.98 (0.95, 1.02)	0.99 (0.96, 1.03)	0.98 (0.94, 1.02)
Work culture score	1.02 (1.00, 1.04)	**1.03[c] (1.00, 1.05)**	1.02 (0.98, 1.06)	1.01 (0.99, 1.03)	1.03 (0.99, 1.07)
Chaos score	**0.96[b] (0.94, 0.99)**	**0.97[c] (0.94, 0.99)**	**0.96[c] (0.93, 0.99)**	0.97 (0.94, 1.00)	**0.96[c] (0.93, 0.99)**

CI, confidence interval; OR, odds ratio.
All models included all variables listed in table (minus stratifying variable for stratified models).
[a] **BOLD,** $P < .001$.
[b] **BOLD,** $P < .01$.
[c] **BOLD,** $P < .05$.

patient care roles (aOR = 1.29, 95% CI 0.81, 2.05). There was no association be-tween being engaged and receiving a COVID-19 booster (Overall: aOR = 0.98, 95% CI 0.53, 1.83). Being engaged was associated with having high self-efficacy in delivering COVID-19 vaccination information for Black participants only (aOR = 1.91, 95% CI 1.03, 3.52).

DISCUSSION

In our sample of health-care workers in Louisiana FQHCs, fewer than 40% of our sam-ple were categorized as "engaged" at work (low emotional exhaustion, low deperson-alization, and high personal accomplishment). Engagement was lower among those in nonpatient care roles (31.0%) versus patient care roles (43.1%). Several potentially modifiable factors were associated with being engaged, including resilient coping, spirituality, and social support. Negative aspects of organizational culture (specifically, chaos in the work environment) and reporting symptoms of depression or anxiety were associated with lower odds of being engaged. The associations between symptoms of depression/anxiety and lower odds of being engaged, and between high social sup-port and higher odds of being engaged, were stronger for those in patient care roles versus nonpatient care roles, while high resilient coping had a stronger association with work engagement for those in nonpatient care versus patient care roles. These findings may provide insights for developing and tailoring interventions to improve work engagement for employees in patient care versus nonpatient care roles. The as-sociation with being engaged for both resilient coping and social support were stron-ger for Black participants versus those who were not Black. Further research is needed to understand whether interventions to change these and related factors can have positive impacts on health-care worker engagement, overall and in demo-graphic subgroups.[23-27] Notably, nearly half of the sample (46.0%) was categorized as "ineffective," characterized by low emotional exhaustion, low depersonalization, and low personal accomplishment. What distinguishes "ineffective" from "engaged" individuals is a sense of personal accomplishment at work, raising the possibility that efforts to foster a sense of personal accomplishment in their employees, particu-larly among those in nonpatient care roles who were more likely than those in patient care roles to be categorized as ineffective, could help FQHCs to increase engagement by their staff.

Only 3.6% of the sample met the criteria for burnout. There is wide variability across studies in how burnout is assessed and defined,[28] leading to a wide range in burnout prevalence: In their systematic review of prevalence of burnout among physicians, Rotenstein and colleagues documented 47 distinct definitions of burnout across the 156 studies using the MBI, and burnout prevalence ranged from 0% to 80.5% across studies. Surveys that were conducted in primary care settings in summer 2020[29] and August 2021[30] and found a prevalence of burnout of 43% and 56%, respectively, are not comparable to our survey, which was conducted later in the pandemic, used the full version of the MBI, and defined burnout according to published scoring criteria. The low level of burnout in our sample may reflect attrition over the past 2 years of those most likely to have experienced burnout, self-selection into the survey sample of those least likely to be currently experiencing burnout, and a reluctance among re-spondents to admit negative feelings about their work or their patients in their survey responses.

With respect to COVID-19-related actions and attitudes, fewer than half (47.6%) had received a COVID-19 booster shot. Although higher than statewide figures for Louisi-ana (as of October 2022, only 23% of Louisiana residents had received a booster),[31] this figure is lower than estimates from other studies of health-care workers.[32,33] Low booster uptake is particularly concerning among health-care workers, leaving these individuals at high risk for infection given workplace exposure, further straining already overextended health systems.[34] In addition, latent vaccine/booster hesitancy among health-care workers may make them less likely to recommend vaccine/booster uptake to those who rely on them for information and advice.[35,36] Provider recommendation for vaccination against COVID-19 and other vaccine preventable diseases is strongly associated with patient vaccine acceptance,[37,38] highlighting the critical role health-care workers play in promoting vaccine and booster uptake for vaccine preventable diseases.

With respect to self-efficacy in delivering COVID-19 vaccination information, confidence in delivering various COVID-19 vaccination messages ranged from a high of 52.4% confident in answering questions about adult vaccination to a low of 25.2% confident in strongly recommending childhood (younger than 5 years) vaccination. Not surprisingly, confidence among those in patient care roles was higher than among those in nonpatient care roles but even among those in patient care, confidence ranged from only 27% confident in recommending childhood (younger than 5 years) vaccination to 60% confident in answering questions about adult vaccination. Notably, respondents indicated the lowest confidence in the 4 items related to pediatric vaccination, revealing opportunities for engaging and equipping health-care workers with information and resources to address this topic. Black respondents were more likely to have received a COVID-19 booster shot, to have high self-efficacy in delivering COVID-19 vaccination information, and to be confident in strongly recommending adult vaccination. Given that Louisiana FQHCs served more than 460,000 patients in 2019, two-thirds of whom were categorized as racial and/or ethnic minorities, including 57% Black,[39] and race concordance between health-care workers and their patients may be associated with some positive patient outcomes,[40,41] these findings are promising for maintaining the progress Louisiana achieved toward overturning race disparities around COVID-19 mortality through, in part, statewide efforts by LA-CEAL and other groups to address Black-White COVID-19 disparities by actively engaging and informing Black communities about COVID-19 preventive strategies.

This study demonstrated an overall association between being engaged at work and being confident in recommending adult COVID-19 vaccination. Other studies have demonstrated an association between health-care worker burnout, quality of care, and other organizational and patient outcomes: a recent systematic review found associations between nurse burnout and patient safety, quality of care, nurses' organizational commitment, nurse productivity, and patient satisfaction.[42] In our sample, the association between work engagement and health-care worker confidence in recommending adult vaccination was stronger for those in nonpatient care roles versus patient care and for Black respondents than for those who were not Black. Further research is needed to explore these race and health-care worker role differences in a larger population of health-care workers, and to understand whether health-care worker self-efficacy is associated with patient behaviors (eg, vaccine/booster uptake) and outcomes.

This study has several strengths, including its timely focus on an important issue influencing the health-care workforce and its ability to deliver quality health care for improved patient outcomes; a statewide diverse sample of FQHC employees; and measurement of a comprehensive set of modifiable social-behavioral factors using validated scales. Findings should be considered in the context of study limitations. Due to the cross-sectional design, causality cannot be determined; for example, rather than a positive organizational culture leading to higher work engagement, it is possible that respondents who are more engaged at work are subsequently more likely to identify positive attributes of the organizational culture. Due to self-selection into the sample and limitation of the sample to one geographic region, results may not be representative of all employees of FQHCs. Participants may have provided socially desirable responses to some items, particularly those related to organizational culture.

SUMMARY

Among Louisiana FQHC employees, resilient coping, spirituality, and social support were associated with being engaged at work. FQHC employees with symptoms of depression/anxiety (versus without) and those indicating a more chaotic work environment were less likely to have an engaged profile. Being engaged at work was associated with confidence in COVID-19 adult vaccine recommendation. Depressive/anxiety symptoms and social support were more salient factors associated with work engagement for those in patient care versus non-patient care roles, while resilient coping was more salient for those in non-patient care versus patient care roles. More research is needed to understand if interventions that foster resilient coping and social support among health-care workers and improve organizational culture can increase work engagement by health-care workers as trusted messengers for COVID-19 and other health issues.

CLINICS CASE POINTS

- Since the onset of the COVID-19 pandemic, there has been increasing concern regarding health-care worker burnout across health systems and its impact on health system functioning and achievement of positive patient outcomes.
- This study took a positive deviance approach to explore factors associated with work engagement (ie, *lack* of burnout) among FQHC employees. Resilient coping, spirituality, and social support were associated with being engaged at work. FQHC employees who reported symptoms of depression or anxiety, or who perceived more chaos in their work environment were less likely to be engaged at work.
- Depressive/anxiety symptoms and social support seem to be more salient factors associated with engagement for those in patient care versus nonpatient care roles, whereas resilient coping seems to be more salient for those in nonpatient care versus patient care roles.
- Being engaged at work was associated with confidence in strongly recommending adult COVID-19 vaccination.
- Further research is needed to develop interventions that change these factors and test if they have positive impacts on health-care worker engagement and patient outcomes.

DISCLOSURE

The authors have nothing to disclose.

REFERENCES

1. Tagliabue F, Galassi L, Mariani P. The "pandemic" of disinformation in COVID-19. SN Compr Clin Med 2020;2(9):1287–9.
2. National Institutes of Health. About CEAL. Available at: https://covid19community.nih.gov/about. Accessed January 9, 2023.

3. Plunk A, Sheehan B, Orr S, et al. Stemming the tide of distrust: a mixed-methods study of vaccine hesitancy. Journal of Clinical and Translational Science 2022; 6(1):e128.

4. Solís Arce JS, Warren SS, Meriggi NF, et al. COVID-19 vaccine acceptance and hesitancy in low- and middle-income countries. Nat Med 2021;27(8):1385–94.

5. Davis TC, Beyl R, Bhuiyan MA, et al. COVID-19 concerns, vaccine acceptance and trusted sources of information among patients cared for in a safety-net health system. Vaccines 2022;10(6):928.

6. Medicare Learning Network. Federally Qualified Health Center (MLN006397), October 2022. Centers for Medicare and Medicaid. Available at: https://www.cms.gov/Outreach-and-Education/Medicare-Learning-Network-MLN/MLNProducts/Downloads/fqhcfactsheet.pdf. Accessed January 9, 2023.

7. Turale S, Meechamnan C, Kunaviktikul W. Challenging times: ethics, nursing and the COVID-19 pandemic. Int Nurs Rev 2020;67(2):164–7.

8. Hayashi AS, Selia E, McDonnell K. Stress and provider retention in underserved communities. J Health Care Poor Underserved 2009;20(3):597–604.

9. Galanis P, Vraka I, Fragkou D, et al. Nurses' burnout and associated risk factors during the COVID-19 pandemic: a systematic review and meta-analysis. J Adv Nurs 2021;77(8):3286–302.

10. Shreffler J, Petrey J, Huecker M. The impact of COVID-19 on healthcare worker wellness: a scoping review. West J Emerg Med 2020;21(5):1059–66.

11. Bradley EH, Curry LA, Ramanadhan S, et al. Research in action: using positive deviance to improve quality of health care. Implement Sci 2009;4:25.

12. Lawrence JA, Davis BA, Corbette T, et al. Racial/ethnic differences in burnout: a systematic review. J Racial Ethn Health Disparities 2022;9(1):257–69.

13. Garcia LC, Shanafelt TD, West CP, et al. Burnout, Depression, Career Satisfaction, and Work-Life Integration by Physician Race/Ethnicity. JAMA Netw Open 2020;3(8):e2012762.

14. Maslach C, Jackson SE, Leiter MP. Maslach Burnout Inventory. In: Zalaquett CP, Wood RJ, editors. Evaluating stress: A book of resources. Third edition. Scarecrow Education; 1997. p. 191–218.

15. Maslach C, Jackson SE, Leiter MP. Maslach Burnout Inventory Manual. 4th Edition. Menlo Park, CA: Mind Garden, Inc; 1996.

16. Health Resources & Services Administration. Federal Office of Rural Health Policy (FORHP) Data Files. Available at: https://www.hrsa.gov/rural-health/about-us/what-is-rural/data-files. Accessed 4/6/2023.

17. Kroenke K, Spitzer RL, Williams JB. The Patient Health Questionnaire-2: validity of a two-item depression screener. Medical care 2003;41(11):1284–92.

18. Kroenke K, Spitzer RL, Williams JB, et al. Anxiety disorders in primary care: prevalence, impairment, comorbidity, and detection. Ann Intern Med 2007;146(5):317–25.

19. Sinclair VG, Wallston KA. The development and psychometric evaluation of the Brief Resilient Coping Scale. Assessment 2004;11(1):94–101.

20. Delaney C. The spirituality scale: Development and psychometric testing of a holistic instrument to assess the human spiritual dimension. J Holist Nurs 2005; 23(2):145–67.

21. Zimet GD, Dahlem NW, Zimet SG, et al. The multidimensional scale of perceived social support. J Pers Assess 1988;52(1):30–41.

22. Dickinson WP, Dickinson LM, Nutting PA, et al. Practice facilitation to improve diabetes care in primary care: a report from the EPIC randomized clinical trial. Ann Fam Med 2014;12(1):8–16.

23. Kreitzer MJ, Klatt M. Educational innovations to foster resilience in the health professions. Med Teach 2017;39(2):153–9.
24. Tement S, Ketiš ZK, Miroševič Š, et al. The impact of psychological interventions with elements of mindfulness (PIM) on empathy, well-being, and reduction of burnout in physicians: a systematic review. Int J Environ Res Publ Health 2021; 18(21):11181.
25. Dincer B, Inangil D. The effect of emotional freedom techniques on nurses' stress, anxiety, and burnout levels during the COVID-19 pandemic: a randomized controlled trial. Explore 2021;17(2):109–14.
26. Sultana A, Sharma R, Hossain MM, et al. Burnout among healthcare providers during COVID-19: Challenges and evidence-based interventions. Indian J Med Ethics 2020;V(4):1–6.
27. West CP, Dyrbye LN, Erwin PJ, et al. Interventions to prevent and reduce physician burnout: a systematic review and meta-analysis. Lancet 2016;388(10057):2272–81.
28. Rotenstein LS, Torre M, Ramos MA, et al. Prevalence of burnout among physicians: a systematic review. JAMA 2018;320(11):1131–50.
29. Apaydin EA, Rose DE, Yano EM, et al. Burnout among primary care healthcare workers during the COVID-19 pandemic. J Occup Environ Med 2021;63(8):642–5.
30. Sullivan EE, McKinstry D, Adamson J, et al. Burnout among missouri primary care clinicians in 2021: roadmap for recovery? Mo Med 2022;119(4):397–400.
31. The New York Times. Available at: https://www.nytimes.com/interactive/2020/us/covid-19-vaccine-doses.html#by-state. Accessed 3/7/2023.
32. Viskupič F, Wiltse DL. Drivers of COVID-19 booster uptake among nurses. Am J Infect Control 2022. https://doi.org/10.1016/j.ajic.2022.11.014.
33. Farah W, Breeher LE, Hainy CM, et al. Who is getting boosted? Disparities in COVID-19 vaccine booster uptake among health care workers. Vaccine X 2023;13:100269.
34. Yaghoubi M, Salimi M, Meskarpour-Amiri M. Systematic review of productivity loss among healthcare workers due to Covid-19. Int J Health Plann Manage 2022;37(1):94–111.
35. Biswas N, Mustapha T, Khubchandani J, et al. The Nature and Extent of COVID-19 Vaccination Hesitancy in Healthcare Workers. J Community Health 2021;46(6): 1244–51.
36. Callaghan T, Washburn D, Goidel K, et al. Imperfect messengers? An analysis of vaccine confidence among primary care physicians. Vaccine 2022;40(18):2588–603.
37. Oh NL, Biddell CB, Rhodes BE, et al. Provider communication and HPV vaccine uptake: a meta-analysis and systematic review. Prev Med 2021;148:106554.
38. Reiter PL, Pennell ML, Katz ML. Acceptability of a COVID-19 vaccine among adults in the United States: How many people would get vaccinated? Vaccine 2020;38(42):6500–7.
39. Health Resources & Services Administration. Louisiana Aggregated Health Center Data. Available at: https://data.hrsa.gov/tools/data-reporting/program-data. Accessed January 9, 2023.
40. Otte SV. Improved patient experience and outcomes: is patient-provider concordance the key? J Patient Exp 2022;9. 23743735221103033.
41. Meghani SH, Brooks JM, Gipson-Jones T, et al. Patient-provider race-concordance: does it matter in improving minority patients' health outcomes? Ethn Health 2009;14(1):107–30.
42. Jun J, Ojemeni MM, Kalamani R, et al. Relationship between nurse burnout, patient and organizational outcomes: Systematic review. Int J Nurs Stud 2021;119: 103933.

Vaccine Preventable Disease and Vaccine Hesitancy

Peter J. Hotez, MD, PhD

KEYWORDS

- Vaccine • Immunization • Vaccine acceptance • Vaccine hesitancy • Antiscience
- Antivaccine

KEY POINTS

- The success of COVID-19 vaccines in saving greater than 3 million lives in North America points to the promise of accelerating new vaccine technologies.
- Several new vaccines for emerging infectious diseases, including respiratory syncytial virus, norovirus, enteric bacteria, influenza, herpes simplex virus, shingles, dengue, malaria, and Chagas disease, may become available over the next 5 years.
- New vaccines for cancer and other noncommunicable diseases are also in development.
- Successful uptake and delivery of these vaccines will require expanded efforts to communicate vaccine safety and efficacy and maintain commitments to vaccine equity and diplomacy.
- This will also require heightened efforts to counter rising antivaccine activism.

INTRODUCTION: IMPACT OF COVID-19 IMMUNIZATIONS

Since 2000, an estimated 50 million deaths have been averted through global immunization programs,[1] including many pediatric lives saved through the actions of Gavi, the Vaccine Alliance of international partners.[2] Some estimates project that up to 100 million deaths could be averted before the close of this decade.[1]

Arguably such vaccination activities comprise the most impactful public health programs in modern human history. Developing and distributing vaccines also represents the top priority in preventing current and future pandemics. There were not many public health victories in the COVID-19 pandemic of 2019 to 2023, but (not surprisingly) among them was the impact of COVID-19 vaccinations in North America, especially in the United States and Canada. Through Operation Warp Speed in the United States, and advance purchase arrangements with the multinational vaccine producers, literally millions of lives were saved by delivering highly effective messenger

Department of Pediatrics and Molecular Virology and Microbiology, Texas Children's Hospital Center for Vaccine Development, National School of Tropical Medicine, Baylor College of Medicine, Texas Medical Center, One Baylor Plaza, Suite 164a, Houston, TX 77030, USA
E-mail address: hotez@bcm.edu
Twitter: @PeterHotez (P.J.H.)

Med Clin N Am 107 (2023) 979–987
https://doi.org/10.1016/j.mcna.2023.05.012
medical.theclinics.com

RNA (mRNA), adenovirus-vector, nanoparticle, and other COVID-19 vaccines. For example, in the Unites States alone, as the first vaccines rolled out in December 2020 and until March 2022, one estimate finds that COVID-19 immunizations averted almost 2.3 million deaths and prevented 17 million hospitalizations.[3] Moreover, the economic impact of COVID-19 vaccinations on the United States economy was profound with almost one trillion dollars saved in direct and indirect health care costs.[3] An update of those numbers extended through November 2022 indicates that the US COVID-19 vaccination program prevented 3.2 million deaths, 18.5 million hospitalizations, and $1.15 trillion in medical costs, as well as 120 million COVID-19 infections.[4]

In 2023, the fourth year of the COVID-19 pandemic, the goalposts have shifted in terms of the number of Immunizations required to prevent hospitalizations and deaths. During the deadly delta variant wave in 2021 in North America, 2 mRNA vaccine doses constituted a full immunization course required to prevent more than 90% of the COVID-19 deaths.[5,6] However, as the virus evolved into omicron immune escape subvariants, it became essential to boost the population with a third or even fourth vaccine dose to maintain similar levels of protection.[7] In addition, a new bivalent booster was required to cross-neutralize the newest omicron immune escape variants, such as BQ.1.1 or XBB.1.5, that accelerated in early 2023.[8] However, in North America, only Canada exhibited consistently high boosting rates, with many nations, including the world's low- and middle-income countries (LMICs), left mostly unboosted. In the presence of circulating omicron immune escape variants, new vulnerabilities may arise owing to such low boosting rates accompanied by waning herd immunity. For example, this phenomenon led a catastrophic wave of COVID-19 deaths in China during the last quarter of 2022 and first quarter of 2023.[9] This reality led to calls for expanding bivalent booster access as the newest means to achieve equity.[10] Therefore, success in defeating COVID-19 may depend on renewed efforts to encourage bivalent booster shots, both in North America and globally.

BUILDING ON THE STRENGTHS OF COVID-19 IMMUNIZATIONS

The pandemic provided proof-of-concept that it was possible to accelerate both new vaccine production and clinical testing, with only a 1-year timeframe between the time Western scientists first learned about the virus emergence until the delivery of the first mRNA vaccines.[11] However, it is important to highlight how COVID-19 vaccine development built on almost 2 decades of coronavirus vaccine work to produce vaccines for severe acute respiratory virus and Middle Eastern respiratory virus.[12] That early work first demonstrated why the spike protein, including its receptor-binding domain, was a promising vaccine target, in addition to the steps required to minimize or prevent vaccine-induced immune enhancement.[12] Nevertheless, the rapid development and testing of COVID-19 vaccines were an impressive achievement, which facilitated the immunization of North American and European populations by early 2021.[13] A parallel success story was the advances in regulatory science by national regulatory bodies in North America, the United Kingdom, and Europe that streamlined the structure of clinical trials and data sharing, or their interpretation.

One major downside of this unprecedented speed and level of innovation was how the new technology mRNA, adenovirus-vector, and nanoparticle failed to reach the world's LMICs, such as those in South Asia or Southern Africa, in time to prevent the emergence of the delta and omicron variants, respectively. Therefore, there must be improvements in vaccine technology equity, even though countries such as India and Indonesia ultimately showed an extraordinary resilience in building their own indigenous vaccines.[14] For the most part, these vaccines used more traditional technologies, including recombinant protein-derived vaccines, with levels of virus neutralizing antibodies comparable to the newer technologies from big pharma.[15–18] This included unique vaccine development partnerships between the Texas Children's Hospital Center for Vaccine Development and vaccine producers in India and Indonesia.[14–18] Now, there are efforts to develop bivalent versions of all of these COVID-19 vaccines to target new omicron immune escape variants and their spin-off subvariants.[10]

For the mRNA vaccine technology, there are several exciting new vaccines under development for both neglected and emerging pathogens.[19] These include new mRNA vaccines for malaria, tuberculosis, and neglected tropical diseases.[19,20] Bio-NTech (Germany) with Pfizer is advancing the development of new mRNA vaccines for influenza,[19] and there are some prospects for a new universal influenza mRNA vaccine.[21] Moderna (United States) is also advancing new mRNA vaccines for shingles and herpes simplex virus infection.[19] This work will undoubtedly benefit from the regulatory precedents set by having COVID-19 mRNA vaccines already pass through detailed review in the United States and Europe, in addition to prequalification by the World Health Organization (WHO).

Outside of the mRNA platform, for low-income countries there are 2 new recombinant protein-based vaccines for malaria from GSK and the Serum Institute of India (SII), respectively,[22] in addition to new vaccines in clinical trials for enteric or diarrheal bacterial pathogens, such as Shigella and enterotoxigenic *Escherichia coli*, and anthelminthic vaccines for hookworm infection and schistosomiasis.[23] Because bacterial diarrheas and worm infections can exacerbate malnutrition, these enteric vaccines might help reduce global hunger now emerging owing to a food security crisis in East Africa and elsewhere. For both LMICs, there are also several different dengue virus vaccines expected soon,[24,25] including a tetravalent live-attenuated dengue vaccine from Takeda that builds on a dengue serotype-2 virus backbone.[26] A new Chagas disease vaccine is in development and expected to enter clinical testing in Mexico.[27] Takeda also has a viruslike particle vaccine for norovirus in development, while other vaccine producers are advancing their own norovirus vaccines.[28,29] From GlaxoSmithKline (GSK) and Pfizer, several new respiratory syncytial virus (RSV) vaccines are expected to be licensed or authorized in 2023 for either older adults or pregnant women (to prevent RSV infection in newborns).[30,31] Finally, active efforts are underway to explore new mucosal delivery routes for the major vaccines highlighted above, including new intranasal, sublingual (under the tongue), and oral vaccines.[32] The new mRNA, adenovirus, and nanoparticle technologies may also accelerate the development of new vaccines for noncommunicable illnesses, including cancer vaccines.[33] Several mRNA vaccines targeting melanoma, lung cancer, and blood cancers are advancing through the pipeline.[34]

VACCINE DIPLOMACY

Ensuring that these new vaccines or vaccine technologies reach all populations and achieve the requirements for vaccine equity will remain a great challenge in the 2020s (**Fig. 1**). In the first 2 years of the COVID-19 pandemic, it was learned that true equity does not depend exclusively on the multinational pharma companies or waiting for new mRNA, adenovirus, or nanoparticle vaccine technologies to filter from pharma to LMIC vaccine producers. Although the multinational companies can have an important role, true vaccine diplomacy will require active engagement between governments and LMIC vaccine manufacturers to produce vaccines locally.[35] This was a rationale for the Texas Children's Center for Vaccine Development entering

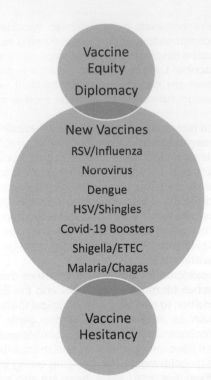

Fig. 1. Introducing new vaccines: the pull and tug of vaccine equity or diplomacy versus hesitancy growing antivaccine activism. ETEC, enterotoxigenic *Escherichia coli*; HSV, herpes simplex virus.

into partnerships with a vaccine producer in India (Biological E) and Indonesia (Bio-Farma) to produce, test, and deliver Corbevax and IndoVac, respectively.[15,16,35] Almost 100 million doses of these vaccines have been administered since 2022. Astra-Zeneca and Oxford University also collaborated to accelerate its adenovirus-based COVID-19 vaccine with the SII leading to the production of CoviShield for India and elsewhere.[35] Lessons learned from these experiences will be crucial for developing and introducing the new vaccines highlighted above. Potentially they could serve as a model for new LMIC vaccine producers on the African continent, the Middle East, or in Latin America.

After the pediatric *Haemophilus influenzae type b* (Hib) vaccine was introduced in the United States during the 1980s, it was rapidly adopted by pediatricians and accepted by parents. This acceptance almost immediately resulted in dramatic declines in Hib-related illnesses.[36] By the 1990s, invasive Hib illness was largely eliminated from North America.

In contrast, since 2000, the introduction of other new vaccines in North America has not always met with the same levels of enthusiasm or uptake. For instance, the Food and Drug Administration approved the first human papillomavirus (HPV) vaccine in 2006 to prevent HPV strains linked to cervical cancer and other cancers.[37] Currently, Merck's Gardasil 9 is the only vaccine for HPV available in the United States. These HPV vaccines produced significant declines in the prevalence of the HPV strains that were targeted by the first version of the Gardasil vaccine, particularly for women in their 20s.[37] However, HPV vaccine uptake and acceptance remain low in some areas of the United States, especially in Southern states, such as Mississippi, Oklahoma, and Tennessee, or in the Mountain West states of Idaho, Utah, and Wyoming, where the estimated vaccine coverage for adolescents is less than 46% to 47%.[37] In only 5 states—Hawaii, Maryland, Massachusetts, North Dakota, and Rhode Island—is the HPV vaccination higher than 64% among adolescents 13 to 17 years.[37] This low uptake remains in stark contrast to other high-income countries. For example, far higher HPV vaccination coverage in adolescents has been achieved in Canada, Australia, and several European countries, and even in some LMICs.[38] Since 2017, 80% of Australian adolescents have received a 3-dose immunization course, through a national, school-based program.[38] Now, Australia's federal government has made commitments to eliminate cervical cancer through accelerated HPV immunizations and other measures.[39]

The factors underlying low HPV vaccine uptake in the United States relative to other high-income countries remain under active investigations. At first glance, it appears that repairing such efforts must be linked to improvements in communicating the risks of remaining unvaccinated,[40] together with information showing that HPV-vaccinated adolescents are no more likely to engage in sexual activity than those who are unvaccinated.[41] However, a reality has set in that the factors discouraging HPV vaccine acceptance represent just one aspect of a larger antivaccine ecosystem in the United States, and one that has since spread to neighboring Canada and even LMICs.[42]

Antivaccine activism in North America accelerated in the 2000s following a report published in 1998 claiming that an immunization with the measles-mumps-rubella (MMR) vaccine for infants could lead to pervasive developmental disorder (autism).[43] Despite the publication of several well-conducted and peer-reviewed studies showing that there was no MMR-autism link, antivaccine activists took advantage of the growing public access to social media by promoting unwarranted fears about this vaccine. Later, the activists would switch up the basis for their concerns regarding childhood immunizations. For example, after initially blaming the MMR vaccine, they subsequently claimed the thimerosal preservative in some infant vaccines caused autism.[43] Then they shifted again, insisting that vaccines were spaced too close together, and that somehow this overwhelmed the immune system to cause autism, or that an alum adjuvant was responsible.[43] However, each time the scientific community debunked these assertions through carefully conducted epidemiologic studies or experimental work performed in laboratory animals.

Eventually, the antivaccine community began pivoting away from autism in order to shift to the introduction of new vaccines. This new tactic began with the HPV vaccine, as antivaccine activists falsely claimed that it might cause infertility, autoimmunity, or other chronic conditions.[44] This was not only true in North America—in 2013, the Japanese Ministry of Health, Labor, and Welfare suspended its HPV vaccine program and recommendations, although the program was allowed to resume in 2021.[45] However, a dangerous precedent was set that antivaccine activists had the power, organization, and bandwidth to disrupt the introduction of a new vaccine.

During the COVID-19 pandemic, resistance to a new vaccine introduction reached a new level. Although more than 3 million lives were saved in the United States through new COVID-19 vaccinations based on mRNA, adenovirus, and nanoparticle platforms,[3] many Americans also died needlessly because they refused a COVID-19 immunization even after vaccines had become widely available by May 2021. In Texas, for example, an estimated 40,000 people lost their lives because of COVID-19 vaccine refusal, mostly during the delta variant wave in the last half of 2021, and the early BA.1 omicron wave during the winter of 2022.[46] As many as 200,000 unvaccinated Americans may have also died needlessly during this period.[47] Beyond the resistance to new vaccine introduction during the COVID-19 pandemic was the increasing politicization of vaccines.[48] Through "health freedom" propaganda promoted by elected leaders on the far right and conservative news channels,[49,50] especially Fox News,[51] vaccine refusal became a type of badge of political allegiance. Americans living in Southern states refused vaccines because they were gaslighted into believing that the COVID-19 vaccines were either ineffective or unsafe, or that they represented tools of oppression.[47–52] This was especially true in Texas and other states where the health freedom movement began during the 2010s.[53] During the second half of 2021 and into 2022, disproportionately the COVID-19 deaths occurred among the unvaccinated in conservative or "red" states, so much so that *The New York Times* simply labeled this phenomenon as "red Covid."[47,52,54] This phenomenon extended into Canada around the "freedom convoy" antivaccine protests of 2022.

AVERTING A VACCINE CATASTROPHE

A major concern for national governments and international health agencies, including the WHO, is how antivaccine activism might now spill over into other vaccination programs.[42] This might have a role in promoting resistance to the introduction of new malaria or other vaccines intended specifically for LMICs.[22] A globalizing antivaccine movement could also extend to all routine childhood immunizations and hasten the reemergence of measles, pertussis, or even polio globally. In 2022, the WHO announced that the "COVID-19 pandemic fuels largest continued backslide in vaccinations in three decades,"[55] with much of that due to the social disruptions from the pandemic, but now even as the pandemic wanes, antivaccine activism could prevent a return to baseline immunization rates. An ensuing decline in herd immunity and a return of measles, pertussis, or other ancient scourges would have catastrophic consequence for global child health, and possibly even begin to reverse many of the successes over the past 20 years through the Gavi Alliance and other international vaccination campaigns. It could also derail efforts to introduce new and important vaccines for RSV, norovirus, dengue, and other major infectious pathogens highlighted above.

Therefore, it is imperative that the major partners of the Gavi Alliance, including the WHO, UNICEF, the Gates Foundation, and stakeholder governments, recognize the dangers of a globalized and politically empowered antivaccine movement. Antivaccine activism has already derailed cervical cancer elimination efforts in the United States and Japan and precipitated the untimely COVID-19 deaths of hundreds of thousands of people in North America—that might otherwise have been prevented. Antivaccine activism has emerged as a potent killing force, and one that requires new and innovative solutions. Because in North America the antivaccine movement now aligns to a political infrastructure, its dissolution may also depend on political interventions, or at least those that might fall outside the traditional health sector.[47] Failing to do so could erode vaccine confidence worldwide.

DISCLOSURE

Prof. P.J. Hotez is a coinventor on vaccine patents for neglected tropical diseases owned by Baylor College of Medicine (BCM). He is also a coinventor of a COVID-19 recombinant protein vaccine technology owned by BCM that was recently licensed by Baylor Ventures nonexclusively and with no patent restrictions to several companies committed to advance vaccines for low- and middle-income countries. These include Biological E (India), BioFarma (Indonesia), Incepta (Bangladesh), and ImmunityBio (United States with partnerships is the African Continent, including Botswana and South Africa). The coinventors have no involvement in license negotiations conducted by BCM. Similar to other research universities, a long-standing BCM policy provides its faculty and staff, who make discoveries and that result in a commercial license, a share of any royalty income. Any such distribution will be undertaken in accordance with BCM policy. In addition, Dr P.J. Hotez is also the author of several books published by academic presses (ASM–Wiley and Johns Hopkins University Press), and he receives modest royalty income from this activity.

REFERENCES

1. Toor J, Echeverria-Londono S, Li X, et al. Lives saved with vaccination for 10 pathogens across 112 countries in a pre-COVID-19 world. Elife 2021;10:e67635.
2. Hotez PJ. Immunizations and vaccines: a decade of successes and reversals, and a call for 'vaccine diplomacy'. Int Health 2019;11(5):331–3.
3. Sah P, Vilches TN, Pandey A, et al. Estimating the impact of vaccination on reducing COVID-19 burden in the United States: December 2020 to March 2022. J Glob Health 2022;12:03062.
4. Meagan C. Fitzpatrick et al. Two Years of U.S. COVID-19 Vaccines Have Prevented Millions of Hospitalizations and Deaths. To the Point (blog), Commonwealth Fund, Dec. 13, 2022. Available at: https://doi.org/10.26099/whsf-fp90. Accessed January 3, 2023.
5. Sheikh A, Robertson C, Taylor B. BNT162b2 and ChAdOx1 nCoV-19 vaccine effectiveness against death from the delta variant. N Engl J Med 2021;385: 2195–7.
6. Self WH, Tenforde MW, Rhoads JP, et al. Comparative Effectiveness of Moderna, Pfizer-BioNTech, and Janssen (Johnson & Johnson) vaccines in preventing COVID-19 hospitalizations among adults without immunocompromising conditions - United States, March-August 2021. MMWR Morb Mortal Wkly Rep 2021; 70:1337-43.
7. Adams K, Rhoads JP, Surie D, et al. Influenza and other viruses in the AcutelY ill (IVY) Network. Vaccine effectiveness of primary series and booster doses against covid-19 associated hospital admissions in the United States: living test negative design study. BMJ 2022;379:e072065.
8. Davis-Gardner ME, Lai L, Wali B, et al. Neutralization against BA.2.75.2, BQ.1.1, and XBB from mRNA Bivalent Booster. N Engl J Med 2022;388:183–5.
9. Bai Y, Peng Z, Wei F, et al. Study on the COVID-19 epidemic in mainland China between November 2022 and January 2023, with prediction of its tendency. J Biosaf Biosecur 2023;5(1):39–44.
10. Hotez PJ. SARS-CoV-2 variants offer a second chance to fix vaccine inequities. Nat Rev Microbiol 2022;21:127–8.
11. Hotez PJ. Vaccinating Cassandra. EClinicalMedicine 2021;31:100711.
12. Haynes BF, Corey L, Fernandes P, et al. Prospects for a safe COVID-19 vaccine. Sci Transl Med 2020;12:eabe0948.
13. Lancet Commission on COVID-19 vaccines and therapeutics task force members. operation warp speed: implications for global vaccine security. Lancet Glob Health 2021;9:e1017–21.
14. Sachs JD, Karim SSA, Aknin L, et al. The Lancet Commission on lessons for the future from the COVID-19 pandemic. Lancet 2022;400:1224–80.
15. Hotez PJ, Bottazzi ME. Whole inactivated virus and protein-based COVID-19 Vaccines. Annu Rev Med 2022;73:55–64.

16. Thuluva S, Paradkar V, Gunneri SR, et al. Evaluation of safety and immunogenicity of receptor-binding domain-based COVID-19 vaccine (Corbevax) to select the optimum formulation in open-label, multicentre, and randomised phase-1/2 and phase-2 clinical trials. EBioMedicine 2022;83:104217.
17. Marchese AM, Beyhaghi H, Orenstein WA. With established safe and effective use, protein vaccines offer another choice against COVID-19. Vaccine 2022; 40(46):6567–9.
18. Heidary M, Kaviar VH, Shirani M, et al. A comprehensive review of the protein subunit vaccines against COVID-19. Front Microbiol 2022;13:927306.
19. Naddaf M. The science events to watch for in 2023. Nature 2022.
20. Versteeg L, Almutairi MM, Hotez PJ, et al. Enlisting the mRNA vaccine platform to combat parasitic infections. Vaccines (Basel) 2019;7:122.
21. Arevalo CP, Bolton MJ, Le Sage V, et al. A multivalent nucleoside-modified mRNA vaccine against all known influenza virus subtypes. Science 2022;378:899–904.
22. Hotez PJ, Matshaba M. Promise of new malaria vaccines. BMJ 2022;379:o2462.
23. Hotez PJ. Malnutrition vaccines for an imminent global food catastrophe. Trends Pharmacol Sci 2022;43:994–7.
24. Zeyaullah M, Muzammil K, AlShahrani AM, et al. Preparedness for the dengue epidemic: vaccine as a Viable approach. Vaccines (Basel) 2022;10:1940.
25. Hou J, Ye W, Chen J. Current development and challenges of tetravalent live-attenuated dengue vaccines. Front Immunol 2022;13:840104.
26. Tricou V, Sáez-Llorens X, Yu D, et al. Safety and immunogenicity of a tetravalent dengue vaccine in children aged 2-17 years: a randomised, placebo-controlled, phase 2 trial. Lancet 2020;395:1434–43.
27. Jones KM, Poveda C, Versteeg L, et al. Preclinical advances and the immuno-physiology of a new therapeutic Chagas disease vaccine. Expert Rev Vaccines 2022;21:1185–203.
28. Tan M. Norovirus vaccines: current clinical development and challenges. Pathogens 2021;10:1641.
29. Winder N, Gohar S, Muthana M. Norovirus: an overview of virology and preventative measures. Viruses 2022;14:2811.
30. Peeples ME. Next-generation RSV vaccines avoid flipping out. Sci Transl Med 2022;14:eade9984.
31. Li Y, Wang X, Blau DM, et al. Global, regional, and national disease burden estimates of acute lower respiratory infections due to respiratory syncytial virus in children younger than 5 years in 2019: a systematic analysis. Lancet 2022;399:2047–64.
32. Anggraeni R, Ana ID, Wihadmadyatami H. Development of mucosal vaccine delivery: an overview on the mucosal vaccines and their adjuvants. Clin Exp Vaccine Res 2022;11:235–48.
33. Gupta M, Wahi A, Sharma P, et al. Recent advances in cancer vaccines: challenges, achievements, and futuristic prospects. Vaccines (Basel) 2022;10:2011.
34. Lorentzen CL, Haanen JB, Met Ö SIM. Clinical advances and ongoing trials on mRNA vaccines for cancer treatment. Lancet Oncol 2022;23:e450–8 [Erratum in: Lancet Oncol. 2022;23:e492].
35. Hotez PJ. COVID-19 vaccines: the imperfect instruments of vaccine diplomacy. J Travel Med 2022;29:taac063.
36. Centers for Disease Control and Prevention (CDC). Progress toward elimination of Haemophilus influenzae type b disease among infants and children–United States, 1987-1993. MMWR Morb Mortal Wkly Rep 1994;43:144–8.

37. Kaiser Family Foundation. Women's Health Policy. The HPV Vaccine Access and use in the U.S. July 12, 2021, access-and-use-in-the-u-s/">. Available at: https://www.kff.org/womens-health-policy/fact-sheet/the-hpv-vaccine-access-and-use-in-the-u-s/. Accessed January 3, 2023.
38. Vujovich-Dunn C, Wand H, Brotherton JML, et al. Measuring school level attributable risk to support school-based HPV vaccination programs. BMC Public Health 2022;22:822.
39. Hayes P. Australia continues push to eliminate cervical cancer. News GP. November 17, 2021.Available at: https://www1.racgp.org.au/newsgp/clinical/australia-continues-push-to-eliminate-cervical-can. Accessed January 3, 2022.
40. Niccolai LM, Johnson NP, Torres A, et al. Messaging of different disease outcomes for human papillomavirus vaccination: a systematic review. J Adolesc Health 2022. S1054–S1139X(22)00717-0.
41. Cook EE, Venkataramani AS, Kim JJ, et al. Legislation to Increase Uptake of HPV Vaccination and Adolescent Sexual Behaviors. Pediatrics 2018;142:e20180458.
42. Hotez PJ. Will anti-vaccine activism in the USA reverse global goals? Nat Rev Immunol 2022;22:525–6.
43. Hotez PJ. Vaccines did not cause Rachel's autism: my life as a vaccine scientist, pediatrician, and autism dad. Baltimore: Johns Hopkins University Press; 2018.
44. Schmuhl NB, Mooney KE, Zhang X, et al. No association between HPV vaccination and infertility in U.S. females 18-33 years old. Vaccine 2020;38:4038–43.
45. Yagi A, Ueda Y, Nakagawa S, et al. Can catch-up vaccinations fill the void left by suspension of the governmental recommendation of HPV vaccine in Japan? Vaccines (Basel) 2022;10:1455.
46. Hotez PJ. The great Texas COVID tragedy. PLOS Glob Public Health 2022;2: e0001173.
47. Hotez PJ. The deadly rise of antiscience: a scientist's warning. Baltimore, MD, USA: Johns Hopkins University Press; 2023.
48. Sharfstein JM, Callaghan T, Carpiano RM, et al. Lancet commission on vaccine refusal, acceptance, and demand in the USA. Uncoupling vaccination from politics: a call to action. Lancet 2021;398:1211–2.
49. Hotez PJ. America's deadly flirtation with antiscience and the medical freedom movement. J Clin Invest 2021;131:e149072.
50. Hotez PJ. Mounting antiscience aggression in the United States. PLoS Biol 2021; 19:e3001369.
51. Pinna M, Picard L, Goessmann C. Cable news and COVID-19 vaccine uptake. Sci Rep 2022;12:16804.
52. Carpiano RM, Callaghan T, DiResta R, et al. Confronting the evolution and expansion of anti-vaccine activism in the USA in the COVID-19 era. Lancet 2023; 401(10380):967–70.
53. Hotez PJ. Texas and its measles epidemics. PLoS Med 2016;13:e1002153.
54. Walter D, Ophir Y, Lokmanoglu AD, et al. Vaccine discourse in white nationalist online communication: A mixed-methods computational approach. Soc Sci Med 2022;298:114859.
55. World Health Organization. COVID-19 pandemic fuels largest continued backslide in vaccinations in three decades, July 15, 2022. Available at: https://www.who.int/news/item/15-07-2022-covid-19-pandemic-fuels-largest-continued-backslide-in-vaccinations-in-three-decades.

Cancer Screening
Patient and Population Strategies

Dorothy S. Lane, MD, MPH[a],*, Robert A. Smith, PhD[b,1]

KEYWORDS

- Primary care • Cancer • Screening • Breast • Cervix • Colorectal • Lung • Prostate

KEY POINTS

- For roughly half of all newly diagnosed cancers, early cancer detection tests have proven efficacy.
- Physician recommendation is the major determinant of patient adherence to cancer screening.
- Reaching high cancer screening rates requires a systematic approach, including measuring baseline screening rates and tracking patient completion of each step in the screening process.
- Cancer mortality racial disparities persist and require addressing social determinants of health; however, cancer screening disparities have been reduced or eliminated by access and affordability.
- System approaches that are associated with improvement in cancer screening rates include patient navigation, having a local champion, and involving the health care team.

INTRODUCTION

In 2023, nearly 2 million Americans will be diagnosed with cancer, and 610,000 will die from it.[1] Cancer is the leading cause of death in persons younger than 85 years[2] and the leading cause of premature death, accounting for 9.3 million person years of life lost each year and an average of 15.5 years of life lost per person.[3] Roughly half of all newly diagnosed cancers are cancers in which early detection tests have proven efficacy.[4,5]

There has been progress in the control of cancer, attributable to lifestyle changes, early detection, and improved therapies.[6] The mortality rate from cancer has declined by 33% since 1991, averting an estimated 3.8 million deaths.[1] However, to reap the fullest benefits of progress in cancer control, greater awareness and action is needed

[a] Department of Family, Population and Preventive Medicine, Renaissance School of Medicine, Stony Brook University, Stony Brook, NY 11794-8222, USA; [b] Early Cancer Detection Science Department, American Cancer Society
[1] Present address: 1593 Deer Park Road, Northeast, Atlanta, GA 30345.
* Corresponding author.
E-mail address: dorothy.lane@stonybrookmedicine.edu

Med Clin N Am 107 (2023) 989–999
https://doi.org/10.1016/j.mcna.2023.06.002
0025-7125/23/© 2023 Elsevier Inc. All rights reserved.

from clinicians, who play a pivotal role in patient uptake and adherence to recommended cancer screening. Apart from system barriers, the most common reason given by those who are eligible for screening but who do not obtain it is that "the doctor didn't recommend it."[7]

Productive interventions can occur at either or both the individual patient or patient-population level. Practice-level interventions include monitoring the patient's electronic health record (EHR) to determine the status of prevention and early detection and emphasizing office policies and team work to achieve greater efficiency. Success in achieving improvement in cancer screening rates usually follows from securing "buy-in" not only at the patient level but also at the organizational level of the practice and the system. Engagement in delivering team-based care with success in achieving screening goals is uplifting to all.

Improving cancer screening rates requires a systematic approach and cannot rely on opportunistic screening, that is, referral for screening incidental to an acute care visit. Furthermore, once referred, many patients encounter barriers and do not get tested, which can go unrecognized. There are toolkits available that provide detailed, evidence-based approaches for establishing office systems and best practices that encompass the full screening process.[8] Although these methods may be specific to a single cancer, the core concepts are similar across all cancers for which screening is recommended, simplifying and facilitating screening uptake.[9]

In the following sections, we will cover prevention and early detection for the leading cancers and recent data stressing the importance of prioritizing cancer prevention and early detection in the clinical setting. We have not included a separate section on cervical cancer screening primarily because it is mostly delivered by obstetricians/gynecologists (OB/GYN). However, since visits to an OB/GYN decline when women are past childbearing age, the patient's screening history must be monitored because guidelines recommend that women and individuals with a cervix can discontinue cervical cancer screening at age 65 if there is a history of technically adequate, guideline-adherent, negative screening in the decade before the age of 65 years.[10] Primary care clinicians play a critical role in human papillomavirus virus (HPV) immunization, which is largely responsible for a decline in cervical cancer incidence rates among women aged 20-24 years of 11% per year and 65% from 2012 through 2016.[1]

BREAST CANCER

There is strong evidence from randomized controlled trials (RCTs) and the evaluation of mature breast cancer screening programs that regular mammography screening is associated with a significant reduction in the incidence rate of advanced disease and death from breast cancer.[11] Contemporary mammography screening programs have shown even greater mortality reductions (>40%) associated with regular participation in screening.[11]

For average-risk women, mammography screening is the only evidence-based method recommended for breast cancer detection. Although clinical breast examination (CBE) was recommended in the past, with greater participation in mammography screening, and improvements in imaging technology, CBE has been shown to offer very little improvement in the cancer-detection rate in women undergoing regular mammography screening.[12] Although few organizations recommend teaching women breast self-examination, it is more common for women to identify change in their breast incidental to daily activities and present symptomatically to the doctor. It is important to recognize that a palpable lump should not be dismissed or passively followed, nor should the clinician find any reassurance if the patient has had a recent negative mammogram. Mammography will not find all breast cancers, and failure to work up a palpable breast lump when the mammogram is negative is one of the most common reasons for malpractice litigation. Digital mammography, including digital breast tomosynthesis, has improved sensitivity compared with the film screen mammography that was used in the 1980-90s. However, the sensitivity of all mammography platforms is diminished in women with mammographically dense breast tissue, and concerns about interpreting a woman's examination as "normal" when some or all of the breast tissue was obscured by density has led to a growing number of state laws requiring reporting breast density on the mammography report.[13] The 2023 update of the mandatory reporting of breast density on the mammography report for all women[14] has led to laws in some states that require an additional screening, for example, with ultrasound or MRI, in women with dense breasts.

Most women in the United States do not undergo regular mammography. Using data from the Breast Cancer Surveillance Consortium, investigators showed only 53% of women had returned to screening within 11-14 months since their last examination, with the remaining (who did eventually attend screening) receiving their next examination after 15-30 months.[15] Successful breast cancer screening depends on high rates of regular attendance. In a recent study, women who attended the last 2 examinations (serial participants) had a 50% lower risk of death from breast cancer within 10 years of diagnosis than serial nonparticipants, but women who missed either one or the other of the most recent 2 examinations before their diagnosis were 23% to 30% less likely to die from breast cancer than serial nonparticipants but significantly more likely to die from breast cancer than serial participants.[16] It is especially important to communicate to patients that *regular* attendance at mammography screening is important.

The current differences in screening recommendations for average-risk women between the 2016 United States Preventive Services Task Force (USPSTF)[17] recommendation and the American Cancer Society (ACS) guideline[18] have largely been limited to women of ages 40–49 years, with the USPSTF recommending individualized decisions about beginning biennial screening (C grade) in the 40- to 49-year age group, and the ACS recommending annual screening in women of ages 45-54 years, with individual decisions about beginning annual screening for women of ages 40-44 years. However, on May 9, 2023, the USPSTF issued a draft recommendation update for public comment that modified their 2016 recommendation by recommending that women begin biennial screening at the age of 40 years (B recommendation).[19] The 2016 USPSTF recommendation that women aged 50-74 years undergo biennial screening remains unchanged, with the USPSTF concluding that the existing evidence was insufficient to assess the balance of benefits and harms of mammography screening in women aged 75 years or older. In contrast, the ACS recommends that women aged 55+ years should undergo biennial screening, or may choose to continue annual screening, and does not specify an age to stop screening but recommends that women should continue mammography screening as long as their health is good and they have life expectancy of 10 years or more. As noted previously, ACS recommends annual screening before the age of 55 years, which corresponds to the menopause, because evidence shows that premenopausal women screened every 2 years have a higher risk of being diagnosed with an advanced breast cancer than premenopausal women undergoing annual screening.[20] The 2016 USPSTF recommendation remains in effect until the public comments have been reviewed and the updated recommendation is published, a process that usually is completed in less than a year. In 2023, the ACS initiated an update of their 2015 recommendation.

Strategies to improve adherence with screening recommendations can differ between those that have at some point adopted the habit of having mammograms, from those who are late or nonadopters, and who therefore may require a more tailored intervention, such as telephone counseling.[21] Apart from lack of access, common reasons for nonadherence to mammography screening include women falling off the schedule due to forgetting when they had their last mammogram, or stop returning for screening prematurely, and the lack of robust reminder systems.

Approaches to targeting community screening efforts at minority populations have been successful in increasing screening rates among Black women and reducing or eliminating the disparity in screening rates when mammography is available and accessible. Strategies for reaching disadvantaged populations include bringing mammography vans to low-income areas.[22] Women with low socioeconomic characteristics who receive care in community health centers (CHCs) have significantly higher mammography screening rates than women in the entire community. This suggests that the CHC health care delivery model mitigates the impact of the social determinants of health on breast cancer screening.[23]

Before mammography utilization reached broad acceptance, a physician's recommendation, or lack thereof, was the most common explanation for why a woman had, or had not, ever had a mammogram.[24] Today, overt reasons for not attending screening include "results of the exam" (fear of finding cancer) and "it's not necessary/have no problem" (no symptoms or no family history), revealing lack of awareness that screening is intended for those who are asymptomatic so that the disease can be detected early when it is easiest to treat.[24] This point should be emphasized in patient education and counseling about breast cancer screening.

COLORECTAL CANCER

The USPSTF[25] and the ACS[26] have very similar recommendations and currently recommend colorectal cancer (CRC) screening for adults aged 45-75 years with either a direct visual examination or a stool test; for those aged 76-85 years, the decision to continue screening should be based on shared decision-making with the clinician, considering patient preferences, overall health, and past screening history. Continued screening of those aged 86 years or older is not recommended because the risks likely exceed the benefits.

Current recommendations include 3 options for stool testing (high-sensitivity guaiac-based Fecal Occult Blood Test (FOBT), fecal immunochemical tests [FIT], and a multi-target stool DNA test [a molecular test combined with FIT]) and 3 options for direct visual examinations (colonoscopy, flexible sigmoidoscopy [the USPSTF additionally recommends flexible sigmoidoscopy alone every 5 years, or every 10 years with annual FIT], and computed tomography colonoscopy). Because colonoscopy is the dominant test used in the United States, a referral to CRC screening has been commonly equated with a referral for colonoscopy screening, and other options are not discussed. However, a sizable fraction of the target population may not wish to undergo an invasive procedure and would prefer a stool test. Inadomi and colleagues[27] showed that only offering colonoscopy to patients resulted in a significantly lower CRC screening rate than when offering colonoscopy or a stool test, which resulted in much higher screening adherence. To achieve high screening rates (eg, ≥80%), it is important to offer the option of a direct visual examination or a stool test, which specifically is included in the ACS guideline.[26]

Modern, high-sensitivity stool testing over a lifetime of screening has performance characteristics similar to colonoscopy in terms of projected deaths avoided and life years gained.[28] Tracking the stool-based testing process is critical to the completion of the screening continuum and answers the following questions: (1) If the test was ordered, did the patient receive the home test kit before leaving the clinic (or in the mail shortly thereafter)? (2) If yes, was the test kit returned and was it adequate to interpret? (3) If yes and the test was positive, was the patient referred for colonoscopy? (4) If yes, was colonoscopy completed, and when? Ensuring follow-up of a positive stool test is an essential role for the practice. A recent study showed that fewer than half of individuals with a positive FIT received follow-up colonoscopy within 6 months.[29] Delays after 9 months have been shown to significantly increase findings of advanced cancer, and failure to follow-up results of a positive stool test is associated with a significantly elevated risk of dying from CRC.[30,31] In some settings, patient navigators have been found to significantly facilitate patient adherence at every step in the process, including overcoming language barriers, providing training and support for performing the bowel prep, securing the colonoscopy appointment directly, locating the colonoscopy suite, assuring receipt of the colonoscopy report, and facilitating follow-up of positive colonoscopy.[32,33] All stool tests are not equal. Only one guaiac test achieves high sensitivity (Hemoccult Sensa), but all guaiac tests require samples from 3 separate bowel movements and are less user-friendly than FIT and multi-target stool-DNA tests, which require only 1 sample, have better sensitivity and specificity, and are not sensitive to upper-gastrointestinal bleeding.[34,35] Clinicians in the practice should take an active role in determining which stool test will be used for CRC screening, and probably it is preferable to have high-sensitivity guaiac tests available to test for the presence of nonspecific occult blood and a FIT test for CRC screening. The practice should also seek to develop a relationship with an endoscopy practice that has a quality-assurance program that monitors basic quality indicators (cecal intubation with photo documentation, adenoma detection rate, ideally multiple adenoma detection rate, etc.) and provides feedback on these measures to the specialists.

At the most basic level, the goal of CRC screening is the prevention of CRC morbidity and premature mortality. With the assistance of the electronic medical record (EMR), the primary care clinician can monitor the screening status of their patient panel, identify patients who are not adherent, and commit practice resources to overcoming the factors associated with non-adherence of screening or follow-up. Finally, it is common to dismiss signs and symptoms of CRC if the patient is younger than the age to begin screening. Compared with persons aged 50 years or older, those younger than 50 years experienced significant delays in diagnosis due to conservative interpretation of sequalae.[36] In a single institution study, the median time from onset of rectal symptoms to diagnosis of CRC was 217 days in persons younger than 50 years versus 29.5 days for those who were older than 50 years.[37] Most new cases in adults younger than 50 years are not associated with a family history or other known risk factors such as high-risk syndromes, inflammatory bowel disease, and so on. Rather than presuming the younger patient with suspicious symptoms cannot possibly have CRC, the clinician should order a full evaluation of the large bowel to rule out the presence of colorectal neoplasia.[38]

LUNG CANCER

For nearly a century, our only effective ability to intervene to overcome the burden of lung cancer has been tobacco control, specifically preventing people from starting to smoke, helping people who smoke to stop smoking, and minimizing exposure to second-hand smoke in the environment. The small difference between lung cancer incidence and mortality rates is a glaring indication of the high fatality rate of the disease, largely due to most incident cases being diagnosed at an advanced stage (66%).[1] The contribution of cigarette smoking to lung cancer, but also cancer deaths overall, speaks to the value of capturing smoking status as a vital sign, performing the 5 A's (ask, advise, assess, assist, and arrange), and checking with people who smoke at every visit for a change in habit.[39]

Two recent trends hold great promise to reduce premature mortality from lung cancer in persons who currently smoke and those who formerly smoked, specifically screening for lung cancer with low-dose computed tomography (LDCT),[40] and novel, tailored therapies based on determination of driver mutations in persons diagnosed with advanced lung cancer.[41] Based on favorable evidence from RCTs of lung cancer screening,[42,43] the ACS[44] and USPSTF[45] currently recommend annual lung cancer screening with LDCT in individuals aged 50-80 years with a 20+ pack year history who currently smoke or if formerly smoked and have quit smoking within the past 15 years. During a shared/informed decision-making process about lung cancer screening, adults who currently smoke should be counseled about smoking cessation.

Because an effective screening method for lung cancer is relatively new compared with screening tests for the other cancer sites discussed in this article, there is generally a lower level of awareness of eligibility guidelines among patients and physicians. Strategies that use the EMR to indicate/remind clinicians to order lung cancer screening are not widely in place, nor are most EMRs helpful in identifying individuals who would qualify for lung cancer screening. To date, the uptake of lung cancer screening has been very low, with national estimates of annual screening among eligible persons still lower than 10%.[46] The important message in this discussion is that lung cancer screening has been judged by multiple guideline-developing organizations to be highly beneficial with a very favorable balance of benefits and harms. System-level interventions are urgently needed to identify adults who are eligible for lung cancer screening, but until they are in place, clinicians must commit to assessing tobacco use history in all adults aged 50-80 years and record these data for ongoing use to identify persons who currently qualify, may eventually qualify, or will not qualify for lung cancer screening.

PROSTATE CANCER

Screening for prostate cancer with prostate-specific antigen (PSA) was expanding in the United States at the time the NCI launched the Prostate, Lung, Colorectal, and Ovarian Trial (PLCO) to determine the efficacy of PSA testing. In 2009, results from the PLCO were published, reporting that no reduction in prostate cancer mortality associated with PSA testing had been observed.[47] Results of the European Randomized Study of Screening for Prostate Cancer were published at the same time, observing a 21% reduction in prostate cancer deaths associated with screening.[48] A novel methodological strategy to reconcile the differences in these two studies was undertaken (due to the extremely high rate of PSA testing in the control arm of the PLCO, severely biasing the findings) and observed similar estimates in the expected reduction in prostate cancer death (25–32%) over 11 years of follow-up.[49] Although it is generally accepted that PSA testing is associated with a reduction in prostate cancer mortality, this observation has not been judged to be a sufficient basis for a recommendation that all men undergo regular prostate cancer screening. Both the ACS and the USPSTF recommend shared decision-making related to testing for early prostate cancer detection.[50,51] For reasons that are not well understood, incidence rates are about 70% higher in Black men than those in White men, and mortality rates in Black men are 2- to 4-times higher than those in other racial and ethnic groups.[1]

The history of prostate cancer screening has been an evolving process of avoiding detecting slow-growing or indolent disease in men who have been screened and have positive finding. The challenge is distinguishing aggressive cancers that must be treated from less aggressive and overdiagnosed cancers, for which rushing into curative therapy can result in greater harm than benefit. In general, there is a clear need for men to have an opportunity to make an informed decision with the support of a clinician, and there are numerous narratives and decision aids to support clinicians and patients in making a decision about testing for early prostate cancer detection.[52,53] Recent data show about 3 in 5 men report having undergone a shared decision about PSA testing and also report that the quality of the discussion is more comprehensive with respect to benefits and harms.[54] If a man chooses to undergo testing, he should be assured that the response to a positive finding is the beginning of additional opportunities for decision-making with the support of his primary care clinician and specialists. More options are available today for differential diagnosis to characterize the aggressiveness of disease, such as multiparametric magnetic resonance imaging (mp-MRI)[55] or evaluation of secondary blood biomarkers (free-to-total PSA ratio, Prostate Health Index, and 4KScore)[56] before making decisions about therapy. If the initial judgment is that the prostate cancer is a low-risk disease, active surveillance is an increasing applied management strategy.[57]

SUMMARY

The burden of cancer around the globe and in the United States is substantial, but adherence to recommended cancer screening has significantly contributed to the decline in the cancer death from breast, cervical, colorectal, and prostate cancers. Many more deaths could be adverted if a greater proportion of the population received regular screening according to recommended guidelines. We are at the dawn of a new era that will bring to bear more patient-acceptable screening methodologies, for example, new cancer screening blood tests and effective personalized precision treatment. It is a perfect time for clinicians in all practice settings to set their goals and implement the proven strategies described here to save lives from cancer.

CLINICS CARE POINTS

- General cancer screening recommendations:
  - Recommend cancer screening to all patients who meet guideline criteria, explain the risk/benefits, and engage them in joint decision-making when there are multiple evidence-based screening options.
  - Track the patient's pathway through cancer screening tests to identify and remove barriers that can halt the process prior to completion.
  - To improve quality, efficiency, and proportion of eligible patient's screened, systematize the practice's approach, including monitoring actual screening rates, impact over time of strategies to increase screening rates, and identifying differences in rates by patient characteristics that may call for targeted group strategies.
  - Strongly consider the possibility of cancer in patients younger than 50 years with persistent symptoms who are below the age to begin screening.
- Breast cancer screening:
  - Low breast cancer screening rates are often due to women forgetting when they had their last mammogram, and patient reminders (electronic or telephone) can be a sufficient prompt.
  - If the mammogram is negative, a palpable lump must still be biopsied.

- Cervical cancer screening:
  - In cervical cancer screening, give special attention to women aged ≥30 years without HPV vaccination and those aged 55-64 years who are no longer visiting an OB/GYN.
  - Performing HPV vaccination is essential for maintaining declining cervical cancer incidence rates that followed immunization.
- Colon cancer screening:
  - Colonoscopy is the first CRC screening test needed for high-risk patients, those who are symptomatic, and for follow-up of a positive stool test.
  - Selecting a high-quality stool test and an endoscopist that meets quality adenoma detection rates is essential.
- Lung cancer screening:
  - Guideline-recommended LDCT screening for lung cancer has resulted in dramatically improved survival.
  - Smoking cessation is the best approach to lung cancer control through primary prevention.
- Prostate cancer screening:
  - In performing recommended shared decision-making for prostate cancer, it is important to reach out to Black patients, who are at higher risk but may not visit due to social determinants.
  - Newer options for workup of prostate cancer are mp-MRI and evaluation of secondary blood biomarkers.

DISCLOSURE

The authors have nothing to disclose.

REFERENCES

1. Siegel RL, Miller KD, Wagle NS, et al. Cancer statistics, 2023. CA Cancer J Clin 2023;73(1):17–48.
2. Jemal A, Murray T, Ward E, et al. Cancer statistics, 2005. CA Cancer J Clin 2005; 55(1):10–30.
3. Howlader N, Noone AM, Krapcho M, et al. SEER Cancer Statistics Review, 1975-2018. 2021. Available at: http://seer.cancer.gov/csr/1975_2015/.
4. Smith RA, Andrews KS, Brooks D, et al. Cancer screening in the United States, 2019: a review of current American cancer society guidelines and current issues in cancer screening. CA Cancer J Clin 2019;69(3):184–210.
5. Wender RC, Brawley OW, Fedewa SA, et al. A blueprint for cancer screening and early detection: advancing screening's contribution to cancer control. CA Cancer J Clin 2019;69(1):50–79.
6. Kratzer TB, Siegel RL, Miller KD, et al. Progress against cancer mortality 50 years after passage of the national cancer act. JAMA Oncol 2022;8(1):156–9.
7. Lane DS, Polednak AP, Burg MA. Measuring the impact of varied interventions of community-wide breast cancer screening. Prog Clin Biol Res 1989;293:103–13.
8. American Cancer Society National Colorectal Cancer Roundtable. Steps For Increasing Colorectal Cancer Screening Rates: A Manual For Primary Care Practices. American Cancer Society. Available at: https://nccrt.org/resource/steps-for-increasing-crc-screening-rates-2022/. Accessed February 21, 2023.
9. Mojica CM, Gunn R, Pham R, et al. An observational study of workflows to support fecal testing for colorectal cancer screening in primary care practices serving Medicaid enrollees. BMC Cancer 2022;22(1):106.

10. Fontham ETH, Wolf AMD, Church TR, et al. Cervical cancer screening for individuals at average risk: 2020 guideline update from the American Cancer Society. CA Cancer J Clin 2020. https://doi.org/10.3322/caac.21628.

11. IARC Working Group on the Evaluation of Cancer-Preventive Strategies. Breast cancer screening. In: IARC handbooks of cancer prevention, vol. 15. Lyon, France: IARC Press; 2016.

12. Chiarelli AM, Majpruz V, Brown P, et al. The contribution of clinical breast examination to the accuracy of breast screening. J Natl Cancer Inst 2009;101(18): 1236–43.

13. Are You Dense. Are You Dense: Advocacy. March 16, 2023, 2023. Available at: https://www.areyoudenseadvocacy.org/dense.

14. United States Food and Drug Administration. FDA Updates Mammography Regulations to Require Reporting of Breast Density Information and Enhance Facility Oversight. U.S. Food and Drug Administration. Updated 03/09/2023. https://www.fda.gov/news-events/press-announcements/fda-updates-mammography-regulations-require-reporting-breast-density-information-and enhance#:~:text=One%20of%20the%20key%20updates,its%20appearance%20on%20a%20mammogram. Accessed March 23, 2023.

15. Kerlikowske K, Chen S, Golmakani MK, et al. Cumulative advanced breast cancer risk prediction model developed in a screening mammography population. J Natl Cancer Inst 2022;114(5):676–85.

16. Duffy SW, Tabar L, Yen AM, et al. Beneficial effect of consecutive screening mammography examinations on mortality from breast cancer: a prospective study. Radiology 2021;299(3):541–7.

17. Siu AL, Force USPST. Screening for breast cancer: U.S. Preventive services task force recommendation statement. Ann Intern Med 2016;164(4):279–96.

18. Oeffinger KC, Fontham ET, Etzioni R, et al. Breast cancer screening for women at average risk: 2015 guideline update from the American cancer society. JAMA 2015;314(15):1599–614. https://doi.org/10.1001/jama.2015.12783.

19. United States Preventive Services Task Force. Draft Recommendation Statement: Breast Cancer: Screening. Agency for Health Care Quality and Research. Updated 05/09/2023. https://uspreventiveservicestaskforce.org/uspstf/draft-recommendation/breast-cancer-screening-adults. Accessed May 9, 2023.

20. Miglioretti DL, Zhu W, Kerlikowske K, et al. Breast tumor prognostic characteristics and biennial vs annual mammography, age, and menopausal status. JAMA Oncol 2015;1(8):1069–77.

21. Messina CR, Lane DS, Grimson R. Effectiveness of women's telephone counseling and physician education to improve mammography screening among women who underuse mammography. Ann Behav Med. Fall 2002;24(4):279–89.

22. Lane DS, Burg MA. Strategies to increase mammography utilization among community health center visitors. Improving awareness, accessibility, and affordability. Med Care 1993;31(2):175–81.

23. Lane DS, Polednak AP, Burg MA. Breast cancer screening practices among users of county-funded health centers vs women in the entire community. Am J Public Health 1992;82(2):199–203.

24. Lane D, Caplan L, Grimson R. Trends in mammography use and their relation to physician and other factors. Cancer Detect Prev 1996;20(4):332–41.

25. Force USPST, Davidson KW, Barry MJ, et al. Screening for Colorectal Cancer: US Preventive Services Task Force Recommendation Statement. JAMA 2021; 325(19):1965–77.

26. Wolf AMD, Fontham ETH, Church TR, et al. Colorectal cancer screening for average-risk adults: 2018 guideline update from the American Cancer Society. CA Cancer J Clin 2018;68(4):250–81.
27. Inadomi JM, Vijan S, Janz NK, et al. Adherence to colorectal cancer screening: a randomized clinical trial of competing strategies. Randomized Controlled Trial Research Support, N.I.H., Extramural. Arch Intern Med 2012;172(7):575–82.
28. Zauber AG, Lansdorp-Vogelaar I, Knudsen AB, et al. Evaluating Test strategies for colorectal cancer screening: a decision analysis for the U.S. Preventive services task force. Ann Intern Med 2008;149(9):659–69.
29. Austin G, Kowalkowski H, Guo Y, et al. Patterns of initial colorectal cancer screenings after turning 50 years old and follow-up rates of colonoscopy after positive stool-based testing among the average-risk population. Curr Med Res Opin 2023;39(1):47–61.
30. Corley DA, Jensen CD, Quinn VP, et al. Association between time to colonoscopy after a positive fecal test result and risk of colorectal cancer and cancer stage at diagnosis. JAMA 2017;317(16):1631–41.
31. Doubeni CA, Fedewa SA, Levin TR, et al. Modifiable failures in the colorectal cancer screening process and their association with risk of death. Gastroenterology 2018. https://doi.org/10.1053/j.gastro.2018.09.040.
32. National Academies of Sciences Engineering and Medicine. Establishing effective patient navigation programs in oncology: Proceedings of a workshop. 2018. Available at: https://doi.org/10.17226/25073.
33. Butterly LF. Proven strategies for increasing adherence to colorectal cancer screening. Gastrointest Endosc Clin N Am 2020;30(3):377–92.
34. Robertson DJ, Lee JK, Boland CR, et al. Recommendations on fecal immunochemical testing to screen for colorectal neoplasia: a consensus statement by the US multi-society task force on colorectal cancer. Gastroenterology 2016. https://doi.org/10.1053/j.gastro.2016.08.053.
35. Imperiale TF, Ransohoff DF, Itzkowitz SH, et al. Multitarget stool DNA testing for colorectal-cancer screening. N Engl J Med 2014;370(14):1287–97.
36. Bleyer A. CAUTION! Consider cancer: common symptoms and signs for early detection of cancer in young adults. Semin Oncol 2009;36(3):207–12.
37. Scott RB, Rangel LE, Osler TM, et al. Rectal cancer in patients under the age of 50 years: the delayed diagnosis. Am J Surg 2016;211(6):1014–8.
38. Myers EA, Fiengold DL, Forde KA, et al. Colorectal cancer in patients under 50 years of age: a retrospectie analysis of two institutions' experience. World J Gastroenterol 2013;19(34):5651–7.
39. Fiore MC. US public health service clinical practice guideline: treating tobacco use and dependence. Respir Care 2000;45(10):1200–62.
40. Jonas DE, Reuland DS, Reddy SM, et al. Screening for lung cancer with low-dose computed tomography: updated evidence report and systematic review for the US preventive services task force. JAMA 2021;325(10):971–87.
41. Arbour KC, Riely GJ. Systemic therapy for locally advanced and metastatic non-small cell lung cancer: a review. JAMA 2019;322(8):764–74.
42. National Lung Screening Trial Research Team, Aberle DR, Adams AM, et al. Reduced lung-cancer mortality with low-dose computed tomographic screening. N Engl J Med 2011;365(5):395–409.
43. de Koning HJ, van der Aalst CM, de Jong PA, et al. Reduced lung-cancer mortality with volume CT screening in a randomized trial. N Engl J Med 2020; 382(6):503–13.

44. American Cancer Society. Lung cancer screening guidelines. American Cancer Society; 2021. Available at: https://www.cancer.org/health-care-professionals/american-cancer-society-prevention-early-detection-guidelines/lung-cancer-screening-guidelines.html. Accessed October 1, 2021.

45. Krist AH, Davidson KW, Mangione CM, et al. Screening for lung cancer: US preventive services task force recommendation statement. JAMA 2021;325(10):962–70.

46. Fedewa SA, Kazerooni EA, Studts JL, et al. State variation in low-dose computed tomography scanning for lung cancer screening in the United States. J Natl Cancer Inst 2021;113(8):1044–52.

47. Andriole GL, Crawford ED, Grubb RL 3rd, et al. Mortality results from a randomized prostate-cancer screening trial. N Engl J Med 2009;360(13):1310–9.

48. Schroder FH, Hugosson J, Roobol MJ, et al. Screening and prostate-cancer mortality in a randomized European study. N Engl J Med 2009;360(13):1320–8.

49. Tsodikov A, Gulati R, Etzioni R. Reconciling the effects of screening on prostate cancer mortality in the ERSPC and PLCO trials. Ann Intern Med 2018;168(8):608–9.

50. Wolf AM, Wender RC, Etzioni RB, et al. American cancer society guideline for the early detection of prostate cancer: update 2010. CA Cancer J Clin 2010;60(2):70–98, doi:caac.20066 [pii]10.3322/caac.20066.

51. U. S. Preventive Services Task Force, Grossman DC, Curry SJ, et al. Screening for prostate cancer: US preventive services task force recommendation statement. JAMA 2018;319(18):1901–13.

52. Violette PD, Agoritsas T, Alexander P, et al. Decision aids for localized prostate cancer treatment choice: Systematic review and meta-analysis. CA Cancer J Clin 2015;65(3):239–51.

53. Riikonen JM, Guyatt GH, Kilpelainen TP, et al. Decision aids for prostate cancer screening choice: a systematic review and meta-analysis. JAMA Intern Med 2019. https://doi.org/10.1001/jamainternmed.2019.0763.

54. Fedewa SA, Gansler T, Smith R, et al. Recent patterns in shared decision making for prostate-specific antigen testing in the United States. Ann Fam Med 2018;16(2):139–44.

55. Kasivisvanathan V, Rannikko AS, Borghi M, et al. MRI-targeted or standard biopsy for prostate-cancer diagnosis. N Engl J Med 2018;378(19):1767–77.

56. Vickers AJ, Eastham JA, Scardino PT, et al. The memorial sloan kettering cancer center recommendations for prostate cancer screening. Urology 2016;91:12–8.

57. Cooperberg MR, Meeks W, Fang R, et al. Time trends and variation in the use of active surveillance for management of low-risk prostate cancer in the US. JAMA Netw Open 2023;6(3):e231439.

Older Adults and Unintentional Injury

Linda Hill, MD, MPH[a], Ryan Moran, MD, MPH[b],*

KEYWORDS

- Older drivers • Unintentional injury • Driving safety • Fall prevention

KEY POINTS

- Falls and motor vehicle crashes (MCVs) are responsible for the majority of unintentional injuries in older adults.
- Clinicians have an important role in addressing risks for MCVs and falls in older adults with appropriate screening and evidenced-based interventions.
- Interventions for fall and MCV risk reduction reducing impairing medications, improving cognitive and physical capabilities, and augmenting environment when possible.

BACKGROUND

Older adults are the fastest growing population in the United States, with the population of people older than 65 years being nearly 53 million in 2018.[1] Unintentional injuries are a significant cause of morbidity and mortality in this population, with car crashes and falls being the major contributors.

Falls represent a significant cause of preventable injury, and fall-related injuries are the single largest major cause of accidental death and disability among older American adults. Approximately one-quarter of community-residing men and women aged 65 years or older, and almost half of those older than 80 years, fall annually, and risk and prevalence proportionally increases as individuals age.[2] Alarmingly, the rate of fall-related mortality has increased over 30% just between 2007 and 2016.[3] Fall incidence is expected to continue rising[4] and carries a considerable financial cost estimated between $30 and $50 billion USD annually.[5]

Fall risk is multifactorial and often the result of the interaction of factors including those inherent to an individual and those external or environmental. Examples of conditions that can exacerbate risk, and that increase with aging, include vision problems, cognitive/neurological impairment, depression, medication side effects, drug-drug

[a] Herbert Wertheim School of Public Health, University of California San Diego, 9500 Gilman Drive, MS 0811, La Jolla, CA 92093-0811, USA; [b] Department of Medicine, School of Medicine, University of California San Diego, 9500 Gilman Drive, MS 0811, La Jolla, CA 92093-0811, USA
* Corresponding author.
E-mail address: rjmoran@health.ucsd.edu

Med Clin N Am 107 (2023) 1001–1010
https://doi.org/10.1016/j.mcna.2023.05.011
medical.theclinics.com

interactions/polypharmacy, hypotensive episodes, muscular weakness, loss of flexibility, and deficits in balance, mobility, and gait.[6] Environmental considerations include home safety concerns including poor lighting but also neighborhood uneven terrain, lighting, and distractions. Notably and unfortunately, a single fall predicts recurrent falls: between 10% and 44% of elderly patients with a history of falls will sustain additional falls. Aside from the significant risk of morbidity and mortality associated with falls, there is likely a bidirectional association between depression and social isolation with fall risk.[7]

This aging population includes a large proportion of drivers; in 2020, there were 48 million licensed drivers aged 65 years or older in the United States.[8] Almost 7500 older adults (aged 65 years or older) were killed in motor vehicle crashes in 2020, and over 200,000 treated in emergency departments for crashes. Older adults have higher motor vehicle fatality rates than other age groups except for novice drivers, and those older than 85 years have the highest rates.[1] This increase in crash rates and fatal crash rates per miles traveled starts increasing at approximately age 70 years. Older drivers are more likely to be found at fault in fatal intersection crashes, with the most common errors being inadequate surveillance, misjudgment of vehicle distance and speed, illegal maneuvers, medical events, and daydreaming.[9] Similar to all other ages, older men have higher crash rates than older women.[8] Older adults have physical conditions that increase their risk of injury and death in a crash, such as osteoporosis, sarcopenia, and comorbidities.[10]

Many older adults maintain robust functional abilities in late life. However, some may experience a decline in visual, cognitive, and/or motor skills, especially in the presence of a disease. Because people are living longer, the number of people with age-associated cognitive impairment and dementia are also increasing. While older patients with cognitive impairment tend to self-limit their driving, a significant number still continue to drive, and dementia may not be recognized by their clinicians.[11] Visual impairments associated with aging include cataracts, glaucoma, macular degeneration, and age-related reductions in contrast sensitivity. While hearing loss is associated with aging, the relationship between impaired hearing and driving safety has not been well established.[12] However, frailty, with the associated sarcopenia, osteoporosis, and reduced range of motion, has been associated with crash risk. Driving performance is usually impaired only after a considerable loss of function since most driving patterns are learned and become second nature. Lastly, the comorbidities associated with aging bring increased prescription drug use, with their impairing side effects. Nonetheless, there is consensus among traffic safety experts that older drivers should be kept on the road as long as they can drive safely. In a large meta-analysis, the risk of depressive symptoms after driving cessation was double, in addition to declines in general health, social and cognitive function, and admission to long-term care facilities and mortality, highlighting the importance of a systemic approach to driving retirement recommendations and the important role of clinicians and health care providers.[13]

SCREENING GUIDELINES

While fall risk is multifactorial, identification of risk factors and referral to/participation in appropriate fall-risk-reduction programs are established as an effective, evidenced-based approach to reduce fall risk.[14] Specifically, targeted strength and balance exercise have consistently been shown to improve fall risk, and accordingly, the Centers for Disease Control and Prevention has outlined an evidenced-based *clinical* approach to identify those at risk of falls to help assess known risk factors and to refer for community-based fall-prevention programs[15,16] (**Table 1**). This toolkit, however, has been slow to penetrate in routine clinical practice, as barriers reported by physicians to implementing comprehensive fall-prevention screening are time constraints, poor reimbursement for falls screening, and that existing toolkit utilization does not easily fit into a Medicare wellness visit.[17] Because of this, only approximately one-third of older adults report being asked about fall risk, and similarly only around a third of those who fall report discussing this with their health care provider.[18,19]

Considerable research has been done to identify the risk factors for crashes, which include, as outlined previously, gender, medications, declines in vision, cognitive function and frailty, and comorbidities. The identification of those conditions most likely to lead to crashes can guide physicians on early management or even reversal of the impairing condition. The American Geriatric Society (AGS) and National Highway Traffic Safety Administration (NHTSA) have developed a clinicians' guide for older driver safety now in its fourth edition.[21] Others have outlined alternative screening options.[22] Health care providers report that a barrier to discussing driving concerns with their patients is the fear of alienation.[23] However, older adults report that they expect their health care providers to provide guidance.[24] A significant barrier for clinician screening is that the current tools available are very blunt in their ability to predict driving safety events **Table 1**.[25]

MODEL PROGRAMS ADDRESSING DRIVING SAFETY AND FALLS
Falls

As noted previously, assessment for fall risk has notable concerns for robust clinical integration. At the University of California, San Diego (UCSD), internal surveys (via Qualtrics, Provo, UT) conducted at an internal medicine meeting of primary care clinicians (response N = 16, 28% response rate) showed on a Likert scale, when asked "Falls are a common problem in my patients," an average of 4.5 (between strongly

Table 1
Office tests to assess for fall and crash risk[a]

Screening Test	Driving	Falls
Visual acuity	x	x
Visual fields	x	
Range of motion	x	
Rapid pace walk	x	
Timed get up and go	x	x
Time maze	x	
Montreal Cognitive	x	
Trail Making B	x	
Clock Drawing	x	
30-Second chair stand		x
Four-stage balance test		x
Orthostatic blood pressure lying and standing		x
Identify medications that increase risk (eg, Beers Criteria)	x	x
Assess for comorbidities	Neuropathy, arrhythmias, etc.	Depression, osteoporosis

[a] Data adapted from the Centers for Disease Control and Prevention (CDC)'s Stopping Elderly Accidents, Deaths and Injuries (STEADI) algorithm.[20]

agree and agree), but when asked "I am aware of community-based resources to help reduce fall risk," the average response was a 2.6, between neutral/neither agree or disagree and disagree; and when asked "I regularly refer patients to community resources when appropriate," the average score was a 2.4, showcasing the need for improved clinical processes. Of interest, shared medical appointments (SMAs) have shown promise in geriatric populations[26] and have the potential to create sustainable mechanisms to evaluate for fall risk within a medical practice. Therefore, a workflow for a fall-prevention SMA was established to comprehensively screen and evaluate for fall risk at UCSD internal medicine, which launched in November of 2021, aimed to provide medical advice and community resources or clinical referrals based on fall-risk assessment. To date, this SMA hosted monthly has clinically assessed 45 older adult patients, and of a subgroup of 33 analyzed individuals, 13 (40%) attended virtually (Zoom for telehealth), 30 (91%) were female, and the average age was 77 years ($\pm$ 7.3, range 64–94). Polypharmacy was common, and the average timed up and go (TUG) was 11.7 seconds, 30-second chair rise 12.3, 27% experienced orthostatic hypotension, and 15% had abnormal Snellen vision screens. Interestingly, we found asking self-report strength on a 0-10 scale was statistically associated with objectively abnormal cutoffs on the TUG and 30-second chair rise, indicating increased fall risk.[27] There is great need to expand and include additional health care members as part of this work and to increase inclusivity for diverse populations including those who have been historically underrepresented in fall-prevention efforts.

Digitally delivered programs are an opportunity that help balance risks and benefits during times of social distancing, improve dissemination, and possibly improve objective measures of function.[17] Therefore, approaches to improve access to fall-risk-reduction exercise, including balance and strength training opportunities, are imperatively important, and growing data suggest digitally formatted delivery may be G Therefore, we developed a fall-risk-reduction program, *Strong Foundations*, designed to be delivered digitally. While there are many such programs currently available on the internet, especially in the time of COVID-19, the novel feature of this program is the delivery of *semi-individualized* instruction in *real* time within a small group setting. This is accomplished largely by the use of the "breakout room" feature on the Zoom platform, where 2-3 trained intern instructors correct form while the lead instructor teaches the larger group. The program was designed with physician input and by exercise physiologists and a doctor of physical therapy candidate, all with extensive training in both group and individualized exercise for geriatric populations. *Strong Foundations* is a 12-week iterative curricular program with three core components: *postural alignment and control, balance and mobility,* and *muscular strength and power.* All the exercises offered over the course of the intervention are appropriate for the target population and are standardized so all participants receive the same basic instruction, but level of difficulty is scaled to participant experience, capability, and musculoskeletal limitations. The program was iteratively designed based on two, 4-week pilot classes with 10-12 participants each, and in 2021-2022, it was expanded for a full 12 weeks across 4 cohorts, with a total N = 38. In this pilot, we showcased excellent usability based on the System Usability Scale (SUS),[28] a nonpriority validated questionnaire which is designed to understand the ease of use of new systems or programs using a 5-element Likert scale. In general, scores >70 on the SUS are considered to have appropriate acceptability of a program/platform. Aside from finding impressive usability among participants, the majority of the respondents found the *Strong Foundations* subjectively appropriate, and attendance was excellent (average attendance was 9.8/12 session or 82% across the entire group). In addition, the research team observed impressive changes in metrics of physical function that were gathered digitally with statistically improved pre-post Zoom-based measures of objective fall risk, namely the average pre-*Strong Foundations* chair-stand and TUG times.[29]

Driving

AAA LongROAD study

In 2015, The AAA Foundation for Traffic Safety funded Columbia University and five participating academic centers (Bassett, University of Michigan, Johns Hopkins, University of California San Diego, University of Colorado) to participate in the largest prospective study of older drivers to date, the Longitudinal Research on Aging Drivers (LongROAD) study. A total of 2990 drivers were recruited at baseline and followed up for 5 years. The study design and population have been described in detail elsewhere.[30] While the final analyses are ongoing with the closing of participant data collection in November 2022, preliminary reports have identified predictors of crashes, citations, and cessation.

Frailty and driving were assessed by assessing falls, fear of falls, frailty markers, and physical capabilities and association with driving outcomes. Frailty was positively associated with low-mileage driving status and driving cessation in a dose-response fashion.[31] Given the known association between low-mileage driver status and increased crash rates and the modifiable nature of the risk factors examined in this study, interventions aimed at improving physical capabilities may lead to an improvement in safety among older drivers.[31] Chronic conditions were associated with reduced driving. Those reporting reduced driving (n = 337) largely attributed reduction to musculoskeletal (29%), neurologic (13%), and ophthalmologic (10%) conditions. Women reported health condition-related driving reduction more often than men (14% versus 8%, $P < .001$).[32] The LongROAD study confirmed the very high use of prescription medications and supplements in older adults. The median number of medications taken per study participant was seven, with a range of 0–51. The total number of medications was significantly associated with a higher rapid deceleration rate. Certain medication classes were significantly associated with other driving outcomes, including central nervous system agents (more speeding events), hormones and gastrointestinal medications (more rapid decelerations), electrolytes (fewer rapid decelerations), and antihistamines (greater right- to left-turn ratio).[33] Dietary supplements (DS) were further looked at in this cohort, given the robust nature of the "brown bag" review conducted at baseline and annually to better understand the total "pill-burden" contribution that DS bring. At baseline, the total "pill-burden" was found to be 7.58/participant, approximately 30% explained by the use of a DS (mean 2.28/participant). Looking across study years 1 and 2, we found that 86% of these older adult drivers reported taking a DS at some point and also found that from baseline, 63.8% continued to use supplements at every point of data collection. Participants who had more prescription medications were more likely to report using supplements as well across the length of the study ($P < 0.001$) and those identified as having polypharmacy were more likely to be on a supplement ($P < .0001$).

In addition, it was found that 542 (18.5%) used at least one potentially impairing medication (PIM) of the 2932 drivers with medication data. The most commonly used therapeutic category of PIM was benzodiazepines (accounting for 16.6% of the total PIMs identified), followed by nonbenzodiazepine hypnotics (15.2%), antidepressants (15.2%), and first-generation antihistamines (10.5%). Older drivers who were female, white, or living in urban areas were at significantly heightened risk of PIM use.[34] Use of PIMs was associated with a 10% increased risk of hard-braking events. Compared to drivers who were not using PIMs, the risk of hard-braking events increased 6% for those using one PIM and 24% for those using two or more PIMs.[35]

Impairing substances are also used by this older driver cohort. Fifty-four drivers (9.0%) reported past-year use of cannabis. Past-year users were four times as likely to report having driven when they may have been over the legal blood-alcohol limit (adjusted odds ratio [aOR] = 4.18; 95% confidence interval [CI]: 2.11, 8.25) but were not more likely to report having had a crash or citation (aOR = 1.36; 95% CI: 0.70, 2.66) in the past year.[36] Rate of alcohol use was also higher in this cohort than it had been reported elsewhere. Of the 2990 participants, 72.7% reported consuming alcohol, 15.0% reported high-risk drinking, and 3.3% reported driving while intoxicated (DWI). High-risk drinking (OR = 12.01) and risky driving behaviors (OR = 13.34) were significantly associated with at least occasional DWI. Avoidance of hazardous driving conditions (OR = 0.71) and higher level of comfort during challenging driving scenarios (OR = 0.65) were less likely to be associated with DWI.[37]

The LongROAD study completed data collection in November 2022, and the final data set has been released. With 5 years of data on 2990 older participants enrolled at baseline, we anticipate additional analyses will shed light on medical, psychological, sociological, and technological issues influencing driving safety in older adults. The project welcomes inquiries from outside researchers on potential collaboration.

Training, Research, and Education for Driving Safety

The Training, Research, and Education for Driving Safety (TREDS) program is a translational community outreach project to address driving safety (treds.ucsd.edu). Founded in 2004, the program has been funded by the California Office of Traffic Safety, the California Department of Transportation, the UC Institutes for Transportation Studies, and the National Institutes of Health.

Clinician Education

Reducing motor vehicle injuries and fatalities by educating physicians and clinicians to better identify impairments in older drivers and take appropriate action has been a goal of TREDS since 2004. TREDS developed a 1-hour curriculum, "Screening and Management of Age and Medically-Related Driving Disorders," to train clinicians to screen and manage conditions and medications that could impair driving. The program, primarily delivered through grand round lectures, has been presented over 110 times to train more than 6900 physicians and clinicians. The program is also available online.[38] Curriculum topics include the epidemiology of older driver safety, methods for screening for medical risks, management and mitigation of risk, reporting laws, and counseling guidance. Risk management is an important component of the training; currently, six states (California, Delaware, Nevada, New Jersey, Oregon, and Pennsylvania) have mandated reporting laws, and most other states have permissive reporting laws. In the mandated reporting states, physicians and health care providers can be held liable for failure to report impaired drivers. On post-training surveys, physicians and health care providers reported intent to change older driver management, and changes in behavior were reported 3 months after training.[39–41] In total, TREDS clinical trainings have reached more than 10,500 health professionals.

Older Driver Education: Drive Safe, Drive Longer

TREDS recognized that education of older drivers would improve self-regulation and driving skills. This inspired the development of "Drive Safer, Drive Longer," a one-hour, interactive program designed to educate aging road users. The class is delivered in-person by instructors at community centers, senior centers, and other community venues.

TREDS has partnered with the California Highway Patrol (CHP) since 2010 to provide officers with evidence-based curriculum, training modules, and technical support for delivery of driving safety programs. TREDS collaborated with the CHP as they adopted the "Drive Safer, Drive Longer" content for their "Age Well, Drive Smart" program. Using a train-the-trainer model, CHP Public Information Officers were trained to deliver the "Drive Safer, Drive Longer" education program across California. To date, over 3400 members of the public have been reached through more than 70 classes.[42]

Distracted Driving

While older drivers are generally more law-abiding than their younger counterparts, unfortunately distracted driving is ubiquitous. Using the experience from TREDS surveys of college/university students and middle-aged drivers, TREDS deployed a survey to older adults.[43,44]

A total of 363 older drivers completed the survey; the mean age was 73 years, and 56% were female. Sixty percent of older adults reported using their cell phone while driving at least some of the time. Participants perceived their own ability as capable or very capable when driving and using the following: handheld phone (40%); hands-free phone (78%); other tasks (38%) while driving. Thirty-two percent of older adults who drive minors reported driving while distracted. Thirty percent of those who were employed felt obligated to take work-related calls. Clinicians should not assume that their older patients are making safe choices on the road and provide appropriate counseling.

Law Enforcement's Role in Older Driver Safety

Law enforcement officers identified the need to increase their competency in identifying medical impairments that impact driving fitness, as well as to improve utilization of reporting mechanisms for appropriate driver re-examination. Motivated by this need, TREDS partnered with the CHP and the California Department of Motor Vehicles (DMV) to address this problem. Law enforcement officers lacked training to identify signs of medical driving impairment, manage the situation at roadside, and appropriately refer the driver to the DMV for re-examination. The TREDS team undertook development of a training curriculum and diagnostic tool based on NHTSA's "Older Driver Law Enforcement Course," released in 2007.

Working with the CHP, the TREDS team developed a 2-hour training, "Law Enforcement's Role in Older Driver Safety," as well as a roadside screening tool, the "Driver Orientation Screen for Cognitive Impairment," or DOSCI, to assess for disorientation.[40] The curriculum covers an introduction to older drivers; medical conditions (eg, vision, frailty, cognitive impairment, hypoglycemia, hyperglycemia) and methods for assessment; strategies to employ during traffic contacts (eg, observation, questioning, use of the screening tool, communication, and referral); use of the DMV reporting mechanism requesting driver re-exam; and community resources for driver evaluation and education.[40] Since the inception, over 5300 officers have been trained.[45] In posttraining interviews, officers stated that the use of the DOSCI tool has been helpful and feasible.[46] Six states across the country (Iowa, Kansas, Minnesota, Missouri, Pennsylvania, Tennessee) and the province of Quebec have adopted the DOSCI tool. The use of the tool was expanded to the DMV/Department of Transportation in the state of Iowa, with favorable results and widespread adoption across the state.[46] The collaboration of the medical system and law enforcement system resulted in feasible and evidence-based management of cognitively impaired drivers.

SUMMARY AND NEXT STEPS

Clinicians play an important role in the prevention of unintentional injuries. Falls and MVC have predictable and overlapping antecedents. Systematic screening for and management of vision impairment, frailty, cognitive impairment, polypharmacy, and inappropriate medications will reduce both falls and MVC risks. Fall-prevention measures, such as strength training, need to be more widely prescribed by physicians and implemented by older adults. Technologically tailored approaches are needed to leverage fall-reduction programs at home, as well as education of older adults regarding home hazards. Physicians need to improve screening and management of sarcopenia.

Fully autonomous vehicles are still at least 15 years away, so both clinicians and their older patients will need better clinical screening guidelines for driving risk. Society needs to address alternative transportation for older adults and improve self-regulation and decision-making support for older drivers.

CLINICS CARE POINTS

- Clinicians need to be more aware of the preventable nature of injuries in older adults related to driving and falls.

- Screening and counseling can be done in clinical settings for fall risk as well as driving impairment related to aging.

- Interventions should address strength, balance, cognitive capabilities and self-regulation.

REFERENCES

1. Traffic Safety Facts: 2018 Data. National Center for Statistics and Analysis, National Highway Traffic Safety Administration, US Department of Transportation; 2020. Available at: https://crashstats.nhtsa.dot.gov/Api/Public/ViewPublication/812928. Accessed July 4, 2023.
2. Fatal Injury and Violence Data. Centers for Disease Control and Prevention, National Center for Injury Prevention and Control; 2023. Available at: https://www.cdc.gov/injury/wisqars/fatal. Accessed July 4, 2023.
3. Burns E, Kakara R. Deaths from falls among persons aged ≥65 Years — United States, 2007–2016. MMWR Morb Mortal Wkly Rep 2018;67(18):509–14.
4. Houry D, Florence C, Baldwin G, et al. The CDC injury center's response to the growing public health problem of falls among older adults. Am J Lifestyle Med 2016;10(1):74–7.
5. Burns ER, Stevens JA, Lee R. The direct costs of fatal and non-fatal falls among older adults — United States. J Safety Res 2016;58:99–103.
6. Ambrose AF, Paul G, Hausdorff JM. Risk factors for falls among older adults: a review of the literature. Maturitas 2013;75(1):51–61.
7. Quach LT, Burr JA. Perceived social isolation, social disconnectedness and falls: the mediating role of depression. Aging Ment Health 2021;25(6):1029–34.
8. Older Drivers. Insurance Institute for Highway Safety, Highway Loss Data Institute. Published July 2022. Available at: https://www.iihs.org/topics/older-drivers. Accessed July 4, 2023.
9. Cicchino JB, McCartt AT. Critical older driver errors in a national sample of serious U.S. crashes. Accid Anal Prev 2015;80:211–9.

10. Traffic safety facts 1998: older population. National Center for Statistics and Analysis, National Highway Traffic Safety Administration, US Department of Transportation; 1999.

11. Valcour VG, Masaki KH, Blanchette PL. Self-reported driving, cognitive status, and physician awareness of cognitive impairment. J Am Geriatr Soc 2002;50(7):1265–7.

12. Dow J, Boucher L, Carr D, et al. Does hearing loss affect the risk of involvement in a motor vehicle crash? J Transport Health 2022;26:101387.

13. Chihuri S, Mielenz TJ, DiMaggio CJ, et al. Driving cessation and health outcomes in older adults. J Am Geriatr Soc 2016;64(2):332–41. https://doi.org/10.1111/jgs.13931.

14. Burns ER, Kakara R, Moreland B. A CDC Compendium of Efective Fall Interventions: What Works for Community-Dwelling Older Adults. 4th ed. Atlanta, GA: Centers for Disease Control and Prevention, National Center for Injury Prevention and Control, 2022. Available at: https://stacks.cdc.gov/view/cdc/124200. Accessed July 3, 2023.

15. Stevens JA, Phelan EA. Development of STEADI: a fall prevention resource for health care providers. Health Promot Pract 2013;14(5):706–14.

16. Sarmiento K, Lee R. STEADI: CDC's approach to make older adult fall prevention part of every primary care practice. J Safety Res 2017;63:105–9.

17. Casey CM, Parker EM, Winkler G, et al. Lessons learned from implementing CDC's STEADI falls prevention algorithm in primary care. Gerontol 2016;gnw074. https://doi.org/10.1093/geront/gnw074.

18. Wenger NS, Solomon DH, Roth CP, et al. The quality of medical care provided to vulnerable community-dwelling older patients. Ann Intern Med 2003;139(9):740.

19. Stevens JA, Ballesteros MF, Mack KA, et al. Gender differences in seeking care for falls in the aged medicare population. Am J Prev Med 2012;43(1):59–62.

20. Algorithm for Fall Risk Screening, Assessment, and Intervention. Centers for Disease Control and Prevention. Published 2019. Available at: https://www.cdc.gov/steadi/pdf/STEADI-Algorithm-508.pdf. Accessed July 4, 2023.

21. Pomidor A, Dickerson AE and Gray SK, et. In: Clinician's guide to assessing and counseling older drivers, 4th edition, 2019, American Geriatrics Society. Available at: https://geriatricscareonline.org/ProductAbstract/clinicians-guide-to-assessing-and-counseling-older-drivers-4th-edition/B047. Accessed July 4, 2023.

22. Dickerson AE. Screening and assessment tools for determining fitness to drive: a review of the literature for the pathways project. Occup Ther Health Care 2014;28(2):82–121.

23. Leinberger RL, Janz NK, Musch DC, et al. Discussing driving concerns with older patients: i. vision care providers' attitudes and behaviors. JAMA Ophthalmol 2013;131(2):205.

24. Betz ME, Kanani H, Juarez-Colunga E, et al. Discussions about driving between older adults and primary care providers. J Am Geriatr Soc 2016;64(6):1318–23.

25. Woolnough A, Salim D, Marshall SC, et al. Determining the validity of the AMA guide: a historical cohort analysis of the assessment of driving related skills and crash rate among older drivers. Accid Anal Prev 2013;61:311–6.

26. May SG, Cheng PH, Tietbohl CK, et al. Shared medical appointments to screen for geriatric syndromes: preliminary data from a quality improvement initiative. J Am Geriatr Soc 2014;62(12):2415–9.

27. Moran R, Ramirez M, Hofflich H, et al. Improving and addressing fall risk: implementation of a shared-medical appointment model in an internal medicine practice. Presented at: AGS 2023; May 2023. accepted/pending.

28. Brooke J. SUS—a quick and dirty usability scale, In: *Usability evaluation in industry*, 1996, Taylor & Francis, 189–194. Available at: https://www.researchgate.net/publication/228593520_SUS_A_quick_and_dirty_usability_scale. Accessed July 4, 2023.

29. Ramirez M, Nichols J, Moran R. Strong Foundations: A Web-based Fall Prevention Program. Presented at: ACPM; 2022; Denver, CO.

30. The LongROAD Research Team, Li G, Eby DW, et al. Longitudinal research on aging drivers (LongROAD): study design and methods. Inj Epidemiol 2017; 4(1):22.

31. Crowe CL, Kannoth S, Andrews H, et al. Associations of frailty status with low-mileage driving and driving cessation in a cohort of older drivers. Geriatrics 2020;5(1):19.

32. Kandasamy D, Betz ME, DiGuiseppi C, et al. Self-reported health conditions and related driving reduction in older drivers. Occup Ther Health Care 2018;32(4): 363–79.

33. Hill LL, Andrews H, Li G, et al. Medication use and driving patterns in older drivers: preliminary findings from the LongROAD study. Inj Epidemiol 2020;7(1):38.

34. The LongROAD Research Team, Li G, Andrews HF, et al. Prevalence of Potentially Inappropriate Medication use in older drivers. BMC Geriatr 2019;19(1):260.

35. Xue Y, Chihuri S, Andrews HF, et al. Potentially inappropriate medication use and hard braking events in older drivers. Geriatrics 2021;6(1):20.

36. DiGuiseppi CG, Smith AA, Betz ME, et al. Cannabis use in older drivers in Colorado: the LongROAD study. Accid Anal Prev 2019;132:105273.

37. Talwar A, Hill LL, DiGuiseppi C, et al. Patterns of self-reported driving while intoxicated among older adults. J Appl Gerontol 2020;39(9):944–53.

38. Training for Health Professionals. Training, Research and Education for Driving Safety. Available at: https://treds.ucsd.edu/hp-training/. Accessed July 4, 2023.

39. Baird S, Hill L, Rybar J, et al. Age-related driving disorders: Screening in hospitals and outpatients settings: Health issues in older drivers. Geriatr Gerontol Int 2010;10(4):288–94.

40. Hill LL, Rybar J. Professional Training Older Driver Safety. Presented at: Lifesavers; March 2022; Chicago, IL.

41. Rajasekar G, Rybar J, Jahns J, Hill L. Mandated reporting of drivers: patterns and preferences. Presented at: American Geriatrics Society; May 2020; Long Beach, CA.

42. Hill L. Older drivers curriculum. Lifesavers; 2021.

43. Hill L, Baird S, Engelberg JK, et al. Distracted driving behaviors and beliefs among older adults. Transp Res Rec J Transp Res Board 2018;2672(33):78–88.

44. Jain P, Unkart JT, Daga FB, et al. Distracted driving and driving patterns in older drivers with glaucoma. Am J Lifestyle Med 2021. https://doi.org/10.1177/15598276211042825. 155982762110428.

45. Hill L, Rybar J, Farrow J. Two-hour training and a screening tool to help law enforcement identify and manage older unsafe drivers. The Police Chief 2013; 80:68–70.

46. Andrade S, Hill L, Snook K. Screening for driver disorientation at the iowa department of transportation, motor vehicle division. Californian J Health Promot 2019; 17(1):1–9.

Women's Clinical Preventive Services

Closing the Gaps and Implementing in Practice

Catherine Takacs Witkop, MD, PhD, MPH

KEYWORDS

- Clinical preventive services • Women • Implementation • Affordable Care Act (ACA)
- Women's preventive services initiative (WPSI)

KEY POINTS

- Evidence-based clinical preventive services have the potential to reduce morbidity and mortality and optimize health.
- The passage of the Affordable Care Act has resulted in coverage without cost-sharing for several clinical preventive services.
- The Women's Preventive Services Initiative (WPSI) continues to identify and address gaps in recommended preventive services for women and adolescents.
- The WPSI Well-Woman Chart and its accompanying Clinical Summary Tables are evidence-based tools to assist providers in ensuring women receive recommended clinical preventive services throughout the lifespan.

INTRODUCTION
Nature of the Problem

Clinical preventive services are designed to prevent medical conditions and identify preclinical disease at stages that will allow for appropriate interventions. Despite the demonstrated effectiveness of a vast array of clinical preventive services for individuals across the lifespan, only 6.9% of adults aged 35 years and older in the United States received all the recommended clinical preventive services in 2019 as tracked through Healthy People 2030, a federal program that sets and monitors evidence-based goals for health and well-being.[1,2] The Healthy People target of 11.5% for this metric has been elusive, with little or no detectable change over the past decade. Additional metrics, including the proportion of adults who get screened for breast, colon, lung, and cervical cancer, have also continued to fall short of the goals set by Healthy People 2030.[1]

Uniformed Services University of the Health Sciences, 4301 Jones Bridge Road, Bethesda, MD 20814, USA
E-mail address: catherine.witkop@usuhs.edu

Med Clin N Am 107 (2023) 1011–1023
https://doi.org/10.1016/J.mcna.2023.06.004
0025-7125/23/Published by Elsevier Inc.

Although system-level barriers such as inadequate access to care and coverage are often cited as a significant obstacle to provision of care, patient- and provider-level factors are also prevalent.[3] Potential patient obstacles to receiving services may include family/work barriers and lack of information or confusion about what services are applicable and/or available for an individual. The inadequate knowledge or confusion is not limited to patients, as providers have also reported frustration with clinical guidelines from various organizations that are unclear or that contradict each other. Further, providers may not feel they have the time and may not necessarily consider provision of the full range of clinical preventive services within the scope of their practice.[4] Providers also may not fully appreciate which preventive services are covered by insurance and therefore may be reluctant to carry out the services for certain patients, who may be individuals who can most benefit from evidence-based preventive care. Discrimination has also been cited as a common barrier to receipt of health care services.[3]

Women have unique health care needs across the lifespan, including pregnancy and menopause-related conditions. Further, many diseases and disorders are more prevalent in women than men including, but not limited to, anxiety and depression.[5] Historically, fewer studies have included women, and subgroup analyses are not performed to determine if certain preventive services and treatments are differentially effective in women and men. As a result, there is often insufficient evidence from rigorously conducted randomized controlled trials to make evidence-based recommendations for women's clinical preventive services, leaving gaps in optimal health care for women.

This article describes the expansion of clinical preventive service recommendations for women, from the US Preventive Services Task Force (USPSTF), Bright Futures, and the Advisory Committee on Immunization Practices (ACIP), to the establishment of the Women's Preventive Services Initiative (WPSI), and will provide clinicians with tips and tools for implementation of evidence-based clinical preventive services in practice.

US Preventive Services Task Force, Bright Futures, and Advisory Committee on Immunization Practices

For more than 4 decades, the USPSTF has been making recommendations for clinical preventive services using a transparent, multistep process that rigorously evaluates the available evidence.[6,7] Recommendations for more than 80 diseases and conditions have changed the way we view prevention, and most clinicians are familiar with and use USPSTF recommendations in their clinical practice.

The USPSTF recommendations are developed for people without signs or symptoms of a specific disease or condition, apply only in the primary care setting or as referable from a primary care clinician, and cover 3 types of services: screenings, behavioral counseling, and preventive medications. Recommendations are assigned A, B, C, D, or I, based on level of certainty regarding the balance of benefits and harms (**Box 1**).[6,7] The process to understand the level of certainty and net benefit and the grading system has been refined over time, but the current procedures and grades can be found online: https://www.uspreventiveservicestaskforce.org/uspstf/about-uspstf/methods-and-processes/procedure-manual.[7]

Similarly, the Bright Futures program, led by the American Academy of Pediatrics (AAP), provides guidance for preventive services and health supervision visits for children and adolescents.[8] The Bright Futures Web site provides several resources to help providers implement recommended preventive services, including the Bright Futures Guidelines, a Periodicity Schedule, and a Coding Fact Sheet, among others. It is

Box 1	
Interpreting USPSTF recommendation grades	
Grade	**Definition and Interpretation**
A	High certainty that net benefit is substantial—offer or provide service
B	High certainty that net benefit is moderate or moderate certainty that net benefit is moderate to substantial—offer or provide service
C	At least moderate certainty that net benefit is small—offer or provide service for selected patients
D	Moderate or high certainty that service has no net benefit or harms outweigh benefits—discourage use of this service
I	Current evidence insufficient to assess balance of benefits and harms—use Recommendation's Clinical Considerations section to understand the uncertainty about balance of benefits and harms

Adapted from U.S. Preventive Services Task Force. U.S. Preventive Services Task Force Procedure Manual. Rockville, MD; 2021. Available at: https://www.uspreventiveservicestaskforce.org/uspstf/about-uspstf/methods-and-processes/procedure-manual. Accessed June 8, 2023.

available at https://www.aap.org/en/practice-management/bright-futures/bright-futures-in-clinical-practice/.[9] All the resources are updated regularly and provide detailed references to help clinicians in their care of pediatric patients.

The ACIP, which falls within the Centers for Disease Control and Prevention (CDC), provides guidance on the use of vaccines to prevent disease in pediatric and adult populations.[10] ACIP recommendations are reviewed and approved by the CDC Director and the US Department of Health and Human Services and then published in the CDC's Morbidity and Mortality Weekly Report. The ACIP recommendations and schedules serve as official federal recommendations, and the recommendations and immunizations schedules are updated regularly as new evidence emerges regarding vaccine-preventable diseases. They can be found at https://www.cdc.gov/vaccines/acip/recommendations.html.[11]

The Affordable Care Act and Closing the Gaps

Under the Affordable Care Act (ACA), signed into law on March 23, 2010, "nongrandfathered" group health plans or health insurance offering "nongrandfathered" group or individual health insurance coverage are required to provide coverage without cost-sharing for specified clinical preventive services requirements[12]; these include USPSTF Grade A or B recommendations, AAP Bright Futures recommendations for adolescents, and vaccinations recommended by ACIP. Although this was a tremendous step forward for health care writ large, there remained gaps in coverage, especially for women. The US Department of Health and Human Services charged a committee of what was then called the Institute of Medicine (IOM) (now known as National Academy of Medicine) to identify additional effective preventive services for women that are not included in the aforementioned recommendations, identify services and screenings that are needed to fill gaps in recommended preventive services, and to explore what processes could be used to regularly update needed preventive services for women and adolescent girls.[13]

The 16-member IOM committee defined "preventive health services" as "measures—including medications, procedures, devices, tests, education and counseling—shown to improve well-being and/or decrease the likelihood or delay the onset of a targeted disease or condition."[13] They identified those preventive measures for which the quality and strength of the evidence was compelling and that addressed conditions with a significant potential impact on health/well-being and which affected a large population; in addition, the conditions include those that occur only in women, are more serious or common in women, or differ in treatment or outcomes for women. The original recommendations, later named the Women's Preventive Services Guidelines, included screening for gestational diabetes; human papillomavirus screening; counseling for sexually transmitted infections and human immunodeficiency virus (HIV); contraceptive methods and counseling; breastfeeding support, supplies, and counseling; screening and counseling for interpersonal and domestic violence; and well-woman visits.[14,15] The committee also outlined a structure and ongoing process for recommending updates of preventive services for women, which ultimately became known as the WPSI.[16]

Women's Preventive Services Initiative

In 2016, the WPSI was established through a 5-year cooperative agreement from the Health Resources and Services Administration (HRSA) to the American College of Obstetricians and Gynecologists (ACOG). In 2021, a subsequent cooperative agreement allowed WPSI to continue to review and make recommendations regarding updates.

The current WPSI Advisory Panel, includes representatives from ACOG, American Academy of Family Physicians, American College of Physicians, and the National Association of Nurse Practitioners in Women's Health, in addition to former members of the IOM's 2011 Committee, a Chairperson, the Multidisciplinary Steering Committee (MSC) and Dissemination and Implementation Committee (DISC) chairs, and co-chairs of the WPSI Pilot Program. The MSC is a multidisciplinary, multispecialty group of representatives from more than 15 health professional and public health organizations. The MSC is responsible for developing and updating recommendations, bringing to the table expertise in clinical preventive health care, health promotion and primary care, critical evaluation of the literature, and implementation of clinical practice guidelines. The DISC is a similarly diverse, multispecialty, multidisciplinary group, developing implementation and dissemination strategies for WPSI recommendations and seeking to create, adapt, and disseminate tools and resources regarding preventive services in general.[16]

The detailed methodology of the WPSI is outside the scope of this document but is available online.[17] In brief, after topic selection, a review and update of the medical literature is conducted by physician scientists experienced in evidence-based systematic reviews (currently from the Oregon Health Sciences University and the Kaiser Permanente School of Medicine), with review methodology adapted from the USPSTF and the IOM Panel on Preventive Services for Women. The MSC then uses the evidence report to develop and vote on a recommendation, which is subsequently released for public comment for 4 to 6 weeks. All comments are reviewed and addressed as indicated, and the final recommendation is submitted to HRSA for review. If approved by the HRSA Administrator, the recommendation is added to the list of Women's Preventive Services Guidelines. Updates go through a similar process, although the literature search builds on the previous evidence review.

Implementing in Practice

The Well-Woman Chart is a unique resource from the WPSI that includes clinical guidelines for girls 13 years and older and pregnant women of any age from the WPSI, the USPSTF, and Bright Futures—all of which are covered with no cost-sharing for all public and most private plans.[18,19] The 2023 chart (**Fig. 1**) includes all recommendations that will be covered under the ACA starting January 2024; the current chart can always be found by clinicians at https://www.womenspreventivehealth.

2023 RECOMMENDATIONS FOR WELL-WOMAN CARE

Preventive care visits provide an excellent opportunity for well-woman care including screening, evaluation of health risks and needs, counseling, and immunizations. *Recommendations for Well-Woman Care – A Well-Woman Chart* was developed by the Women's Preventive Services Initiative (WPSI). The Well-Woman Chart outlines preventive services recommended by the WPSI, U.S. Preventive Services Task Force (USPSTF), and Bright Futures based on age, health status, and risk factors. Additional recommendations for immunizations are provided in a separate table from the Advisory Committee on Immunization Practices. Clinical practice considerations, risk assessment methods, and the age and frequency to deliver services are described in the Clinical Summary Tables that accompany the chart.

The Well-Woman Chart provides a framework for incorporating preventive health services for women into clinical practice. These services may be completed at a single visit or as part of a series of visits that take place over time. This information is designed as an educational resource to aid clinicians in providing preventive health services for women, and use of this information is voluntary. This information should not be considered as inclusive of all proper treatments or methods of care or as a statement of the standard of care. It is not intended to substitute for the independent professional judgment of the treating clinician. Variations in practice may be warranted when, in the reasonable judgment of the treating clinician, such course of action is indicated by the condition of the patient, limitations of available resources, or advances in knowledge or technology. While every effort is made to present accurate and reliable information, this publication is provided "as is" without any guarantees or warranties of accuracy, reliability, or otherwise, either express or implied. The Chart and Tables are updated annually. The WPSI website (www.womenspreventivehealth.org) has the most up-to-date version of the Chart and Clinical Summary Tables.

HEALTH CARE SERVICES	AGE (Years)						
	13–17¹	18–21¹	22–39	40–49	50–64	65–75	>75
❤ **GENERAL HEALTH**							
Alcohol use screening & counseling	●	●	●	●	●	●	●
Anxiety screening	●	●	●	●	●	●	●
Blood pressure screening	●	●	●	●	●	●	●
Contraception and contraceptive care	●	●	●	●	○		
Depression screening	●	●	●	●	●	●	●
Diabetes screening²	○	○	○	○	○	○	○
Fall prevention							●
Folic acid supplementation³	○	●	●	●	○		
Healthy diet & activity counseling⁴		○	○	○	○	○	○
Interpersonal & domestic violence screening	●	●	●	●	●	●	●
Lipid screening⁵	○	○	○	●	●	●	●
Obesity prevention				●	●50–60		
Obesity screening & counseling	●	●	●	●	●	●	●
Osteoporosis screening⁶					○	●	●
Statin use to prevent CVD⁷				○	○	○	
Substance use screening & assessment	●	●	●	●	●	●	●
Tobacco screening & counseling	●	●	●	●	●	●	●
Urinary incontinence screening⁸	○	●	●	●	●	●	●
⚕ **INFECTIOUS DISEASES**							
Gonorrhea & chlamydia screening⁹	●	●	●≤24 ○>24	○	○	○	○
Hepatitis B screening¹⁰	○	○	○	○	○	○	○
Hepatitis C screening (at least once)¹¹	○	●	●	●	●	●	●≤80
HIV preexposure prophylaxis¹²	○	○	○	○	○	○	○
HIV risk assessment	●	●	●	●	●	●	●
HIV screening (at least once)	●>15	●	●	●	●	○	○
Immunizations¹³	●	●	●	●	●	●	●
STI prevention counseling¹⁴	●	●	○	○	○	○	○
Syphilis screening¹⁵	○	○	○	○	○	○	○
Tuberculosis screening¹⁶	○	○	○	○	○	○	○
✝ **CANCER**							
Breast cancer screening¹⁷				○	●	●	○
Cervical cancer screening		●>21	●	●	●	●≤65	
Colorectal cancer screening				●45–49	●	●	
Lung cancer screening¹⁹					○	○	○≤80
Medications to reduce breast cancer risk¹⁹				○	○	○	○
Risk assessment for BRCA1/2 genetic counseling & testing		●	●	●	●	●	●
Skin cancer counseling²⁰	○	○	○≤24				

Recommendations for services from the WPSI and the USPSTF for preventive services for pregnant and postpartum women are also provided in the Well-Woman Chart. Comprehensive recommendations for pregnant and postpartum women can be found in ACOG's practice guidelines and other educational materials.

PREVENTION SERVICES for pregnancy and postpartum provided in addition to age-based services listed in the previous chart	
⚭ **PREGNANCY**	
Anxiety screening	●
Bacteriuria screening	●
Breastfeeding counseling, services & supplies	●
Contraception and contraceptive care	●
Depression screening & preventive interventions²¹	●
Diabetes screening²²	●
Folic acid supplementation	●
Gonorrhea & chlamydia screening	●
Healthy weight gain counseling	●
Hepatitis B screening	●
HIV screening (each pregnancy)	●
Interpersonal & domestic violence screening	●
Preeclampsia prevention with low-dose aspirin²³	○
Preeclampsia screening	●
Rh(D) blood typing	●
Substance use screening & assessment	●
Syphilis screening	●
Tobacco screening & counseling	●

PREVENTION SERVICES for pregnancy and postpartum provided in addition to age-based services listed in the previous chart	
⚭ **POSTPARTUM**	
Anxiety screening	●
Breastfeeding counseling, services & supplies	●
Contraception and contraceptive care	●
Depression screening & preventive interventions²¹	●
Diabetes screening²⁴	○
Folic acid supplementation	●
Interpersonal & domestic violence screening	●
Substance use screening & assessment	●
Tobacco screening & counseling	●

KEY:
● Recommended by the USPSTF (A or B rating), WPSI, or Bright Futures
○ Recommended for selected groups

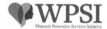
WPSI
Women's Preventive Services Initiative

MEMBERS OF THE ADVISORY PANEL SUPPORT THE WPSI

AMERICAN ACADEMY OF FAMILY PHYSICIANS
STRONG MEDICINE FOR AMERICA

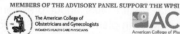
The American College of Obstetricians and Gynecologists
WOMEN'S HEALTH CARE PHYSICIANS

ACP
American College of Physicians
Leading Internal Medicine, Improving Lives

NPWH
NURSE PRACTITIONERS IN WOMEN'S HEALTH
Caring for Women

Fig. 1. The 2023 WPSI Well-Woman Chart, including recommendations for well-woman care from the USPSTF, WPSI, and Bright Futures. (Reprinted with permission from Women's Preventive Services Initiative. Recommendations for well-woman care – a well-woman chart. Washington, DC: ACOG Foundation; 2023. Available at: https://149858107.v2.pressablecdn.com/wp-content/uploads/FINAL_WPSI_WWC_11x17_2023.pdf. Retrieved April 25, 2023.)

org/wellwomanchart/.[19] Detailed information for each recommendation in the Well-Woman Chart is provided in accompanying Clinical Summary Tables that can be found at the same link.[20] The tables include the rationale for the preventive service recommendation, each of the existing recommendations from USPSTF, WPSI, or Bright Futures. Most (n = 27) recommendations on a given topic are from a single organization, but 11 include recommendations from 2, and 1 includes recommendations from all 3 organizations.[20]

One of the obstacles that clinicians often cite for not performing clinical preventive services is that recommendations differ between guideline-producing bodies. In the case of the Well-Woman Chart, each covered recommendation for a given topic is included in the Clinical Summary Tables, but if there are differences in age range or coverage, the recommendation that is applied within the Chart is the most comprehensive, and the language used is that from that particular recommendation.

To demonstrate how a WPSI recommendation is translated into the Well-Woman Chart and the Clinical Summary Tables, the authors take a look at a recent recommendation from WPSI—screening for anxiety in adolescent and adult women[21,22]—and how it is presented in a Clinical Summary Table (**Table 1**). The rationale statement briefly provides information about any relevant background (eg, definition and description of disorder of interest) as well as the current epidemiology and why this recommendation was developed by the WPSI (ie, the most frequent mental health disorders in the United States and rates in women are higher than in men). Finally, an abridged version of the recommendation statement is included: "Screen for anxiety in adolescent and adult women age 13 and older, including those who are pregnant or postpartum. Given the high prevalence of anxiety disorders, lack of recognition in clinical practice, and multiple problems associated with untreated anxiety, clinicians should consider screening women who have not been recently screened."[23]

Clinical considerations are then provided in tabular form. The ages and frequency, if applicable, are clearly stated, in this case, 13 years of age or older, although the optimal screening intervals are unknown. The table then provides a brief version of implementation considerations, highlighting that anxiety frequently co-occurs with depression and therefore screening simultaneously for both may provide some efficiencies in the clinical setting. For this recommendation, screening tools that screen for both are included in the clinical considerations section. WPSI does suggest that screening should be implemented together with team-based approaches in order that effective treatment and follow-up are possible. If a risk assessment is necessary, that is also called out in the table; in this case, universal screening of all women older than 13 years is recommended. Finally, the citation for the published recommendation[21] and the link to the recommendation on the WPSI Web site is included.[22]

For those clinicians interested in learning more about the evidence supporting the recommendation, the Web site includes the link to the systematic review performed for the recommendation.[23] Finally, on the WPSI recommendation page, clinicians can also find a resource developed by the WPSI Dissemination and Implementation Committee: How I Practice videos.[22] For example, in the How I Practice: Screening for Anxiety video, an expert in mental health talks about prevalence of anxiety in the US population and some tips on how to implement the WPSI recommendation in practice.

As mentioned, discerning the nuances between recommendations from different organizations can be a challenge for providers as well as patients. To demonstrate how the Well-Woman Chart can mitigate this issue for providers, we look at the Clinical Summary Table for the single recommendation that includes recommendations from USPSTF, WPSI, and Bright Futures: Human Immunodeficiency Virus Preexposure Screening & Risk Assessment (**Table 2**). In this case, all 3 organizations

Table 1
The clinical summary table for anxiety screening recommendation to accompany the 2023 WPSI Well-Woman Chart

Anxiety Screening

Rationale: anxiety disorders include several related conditions characterized by excessive, uncontrollable worry. They are the most frequent mental health disorders in the general US population; and prevalence rates are higher in women than men, with approximately 40% of women experiencing anxiety disorders during their lifetimes. Anxiety is a common manifestation of posttraumatic stress disorder, stress, bullying, sexual harassment and assault, and other experiences common in women and is associated with depression and substance abuse.

WPSI Recommendation: screen for anxiety in adolescent and adult women age 13 y and older, including those who are pregnant or postpartum. Given the high prevalence of anxiety disorders, lack of recognition in clinical practice, and multiple problems associated with untreated anxiety, clinicians should consider screening women who have not been recently screened.

USPSTF Recommendation: the USPSTF recommends screening for anxiety in children and adolescents aged 8 to 18 y.

Ages and Frequency	≥ 13 y; optimal screening intervals are unknown and clinical judgement should be used to determine screening frequency
Clinical Practice	Consider screening for anxiety in conjunction with screening for depression, which is already recommended, because of their frequent co-occurrence. Validated instruments that screen simultaneously for both disorders may be clinically efficient in practice settings (eg, Patient Health Questionnaire and the Hospital Anxiety and Depression Scale, among others). When screening suggests the presence of anxiety, further evaluation is necessary to establish the diagnosis and determine appropriate treatment. Screening should ideally be implemented in conjunction with collaborative and team-based approaches to ensure accurate diagnosis, effective treatment, and appropriate follow-up.
Risk Assessment	All women are susceptible to anxiety, and universal screening is recommended.
References	• Gregory KD, Chelmow D, Nelson HD, et al. Screening for anxiety in adolescent and adult women: a recommendation from the Women's Preventive Services Initiative. Ann Intern Med. 2020; 173:48-56. https://doi.org/10.7326/M20-0580. PMID: 32510990. • Women's Preventive Services Initiative. Screening for Anxiety. https://www.womenspreventivehealth.org/recommendations/screening-for-anxiety/. • US Preventive Services Task Force. Screening for anxiety in children and adolescents: US Preventive Services Task Force recommendation statement. JAMA. 2022; 328:1438 1444. • Bright Futures/AAP Recommendations for Preventive Pediatric Health Care (Periodicity Schedule) https://downloads.aap.org/AAP/PDF/periodicity_schedule.pdf?_ga=2.90295442.924462059.1671580996-606362568.1671580995. Accessed December 19, 2022.

Reprinted with permission from Women's Preventive Services Initiative. Recommendations for well-woman care: clinical summary tables. Washington, DC: ACOG Foundation; 2023. Available at: https://149858107.v2.pressablecdn.com/wp-content/uploads/FINAL_WPSI_ClinicalSummaryTables_2023.pdf. Retrieved April 25, 2023.

recommend screening all women who are 15 years of age or older at least once. All 3 also mention a risk assessment, and therefore, the Clinical Summary Table also includes risk assessment. References are included for both the USPSTF recommendation[24] and the link to the WPSI recommendation and evidence review.[25]

Table 2
The clinical summary table for human immunodeficiency virus preexposure screening and risk assessment to accompany the 2023 WPSI Well-Woman Chart

Human Immunodeficiency Virus Preexposure Risk Assessment & Screening	
Rationale: screening for human immunodeficiency virus (HIV) infection detects individuals who are unaware of their infection and would otherwise miss the opportunity to benefit from early therapy that can reduce serious AIDS-related events and death as well as disease transmission.	
USPSTF Recommendation: screen for HIV infection in adolescents and adults aged 15 to 65 y and younger adolescents and older adults who are at increased risk of infection. Screen during pregnancy, including when presenting in labor or at delivery, and HIV status is unknown.	
WPSI Recommendation: prevention education and risk assessment for HIV infection in adolescents and adults at least annually throughout the lifespan. Test all women for HIV at least once during their lifetimes, and all pregnant women on initiation of prenatal care with retesting during pregnancy based on risk factors.	
Bright Futures Recommendation: screen once between the ages of 15 and 18 y; retest annually if increased risk (sexually active, injection drug use, tested for other STIs).	
Ages and Frequency	>15 y; appropriate or optimal time intervals or strategies for repeat HIV screening are not known. Earlier or additional screening should be based on risk, and rescreening annually or more often may be appropriate beginning at age 13 y for adolescent and adult women with an increased risk of HIV infection. Repeat screening is reasonable for individuals known to be at increased risk of HIV infection or live or receive medical care in a high-prevalence setting, such as a sexually transmitted disease clinic.
Clinical Practice	This recommendation refers to routine HIV screening, which is different from incident-based or exposure-based HIV testing. Annual or more frequent HIV testing is recommended for women who are high-risk. Screening is recommended for all pregnant women on initiation of prenatal care with retesting during pregnancy based on risk factors. Rapid HIV testing is recommended for pregnant women who present in active labor with an undocumented HIV status.
Risk Assessment	Risk factors include injection drug use; unprotected vaginal or anal intercourse; multiple sexual partners; new sexual relationship; sexual partners who are HIV-infected, bisexual, or injection drug users; exchanging sex for drugs or money; victim of sex trafficking; incarceration; other STIs.
References	• US Preventive Services Task Force. Screening for HIV infection: US Preventive Services Task Force recommendation statement. JAMA 2019;321(23):2326-2336. https://doi.org/10.1001/jama.2019.6587. PMID: 31184701. • Women's Preventive Services Initiative. Screening for Human Immunodeficiency Virus Infection. https://www.womenspreventivehealth.org/recommendations/human-immunodeficiency-virus-infection/. Published January 7, 2022. Accessed December 19, 2022.

Abbreviation: STIs, sexually transmitted infections.

Reprinted with permission from Women's Preventive Services Initiative. Recommendations for well-woman care: clinical summary tables. Washington, DC: ACOG Foundation; 2023. Available at: https://149858107.v2.pressablecdn.com/wp-content/uploads/FINAL_WPSI_ClinicalSummaryTables_2023.pdf. Retrieved April 25, 2023.

Case Study

The following case study places you in the role of a primary care physician. Let us look at how the WPSI Well-Woman Chart can be used to address recommended clinical preventive services for a fictional patient.

A 23-year-old patient presents to you with the chief complaint of upper respiratory symptoms 3 months after delivering her first child, a healthy male infant, via normal spontaneous vaginal delivery. Her pregnancy was complicated by diagnoses of gestational diabetes and preeclampsia. She had been unable to follow-up with her obstetrician for her postpartum visit, as she had to return to work 6 weeks after delivery, but her current symptoms have kept her out of work and she is now seeking care. She had nursed until she went back to work but now exclusively bottle feeds her baby. She and her partner are using condoms for contraception. Her pregnancy was unplanned, and she is not currently interested in getting pregnant.

You address her upper respiratory symptoms expeditiously but recognize that you should try to take advantage of this opportunity to complete some recommended clinical preventive services for this patient. Using the Well-Woman Chart, you identify several preventive services recommended for postpartum patients, including (in order on the chart) the following: anxiety screening, contraceptive counseling and care if indicated, depression screening, folic acid supplementation, interpersonal and domestic violence screening, substance use screening and treatment if indicated, and tobacco screening and counseling. Further, given the patient's personal history of gestational diabetes, the provider recognizes the need for diabetes screening.

You next scan the general health recommendations and identify a few additional recommended services, including alcohol use screening, blood pressure screening, obesity screening, and urinary incontinence screening.

You move to the infectious diseases and cancer sections of the chart. On reviewing the patient's electronic health record, you see she had cervical cancer screening and gonorrhea and chlamydia screening when she first learned she was pregnant, about 14 months ago. She also had hepatitis and HIV testing and syphilis screening while pregnant. All of these test results were normal, and she reports she has been in this same monogamous relationship for 3 years.

During her intake, the patient had denied using tobacco or other substances. The Alcohol Use Disorders Identification Test-Consumption score,[26] which is done for all patients in your office, was negative (scored 2). She reported she lived with her partner at home and screened negative on the HITS domestic violence screening tool, in which she was asked about how often her partner hurts, insults, threatens with harm, or screams or curses at her.[27] Family history was negative for breast, ovarian, uterine cancers. Her blood pressure was normal, and her body mass index (BMI) was 29.

Recognizing that this patient will have difficulty returning for a follow-up visit, you ask her if she would like to complete all the additional required screenings today. She agrees.

Although her BMI is in the overweight range, she does not have additional risk factors for cardiovascular disease. You see from the medical record that her prepregnancy BMI was 26; she reports she is trying to return to her prepregnancy weight. She reports she has been trying to eat a healthier diet and has started walking to and from work when she has the time. However, she is concerned about being able to maintain or lose weight. You encourage her ongoing efforts, offer some online resources, and let her know you will continue to monitor when she returns for future appointments.

Your clinic does not routinely screen for anxiety or depression at intake, but after reading the evidence tables for the Well-Woman Chart, you conduct the 4-question Patient Health Questionnaire-4.[28,29] She scores a 1 in the anxiety subscale (GAD-2) and a 2 in the depression subscale (PHQ-2), both of which are considered negative. You inform her that this negative screening test does not mean anxiety and depression are not present but that the likelihood is low. You also let her know she should reach out if she is experiencing symptoms of anxiety or depression in the future.

You use the Actionable Bladder Symptoms Screener (an 8-item Likert scale tool that asks about frequency, leakage, urgency, and nighttime voids as well as impact on the quality of life) to screen the patient for urinary incontinence.[30,31] She scores a 2 on the Screener (negative screen) and does not have any additional concerns regarding urinary symptoms.

The patient resumed menstruating after she discontinued nursing and is currently on her period. You discuss the full range of contraceptive options with her using a model of shared decision-making that you had seen on the How I Practice video on the WPSI Web site. She has no contraindications to any methods, and, after discussing her values and preferences around all of the options, she decides she would like to proceed with a progesterone intrauterine device (IUD). She says she would prefer to return for that on another day and so you ensure she is scheduled for IUD placement within the week before she leaves the clinic.

You tell the patient that, given her diagnosis of gestational diabetes in pregnancy, she is at increased risk of developing type 2 diabetes in the future. You explain to her that it is recommended that she be screened for diabetes as soon as she is able and, even if negative, that she be rescreened at least every 3 years. You offer to order the test today, but the patient says she will have more time to do it on the day she returns for her IUD placement.

You also order a urine gonorrhea and chlamydia screen that she can also do while she is in the laboratory next week. You explain to her that this is a routine screening test for someone of her age. Finally, the patient had been taking prenatal vitamins while nursing but had run out. You order folic acid for her, given the recommendation to take a daily supplement of 0.4 to 0.8 mg (400–800 µg) of folic acid.

The patient expresses some concern about the cost of the laboratory tests and the folic acid, but you assure her that these are covered without any cost-sharing. After she leaves, you use the online WPSI Coding Guide (https://www.women spreventivehealth.org/wpsi-coding-guide/) to complete your billing for the visit.[32]

Although this case study demonstrates how most of the recommended clinical preventive services for a particular patient can be offered and even completed in a single visit, some clinical scenarios or environments may not support this. It is important to note that these services can also be accomplished in a series of visits over time, but equally salient is that, due to extensive variation in individual patient circumstances and structural and social determinants of health, it may be difficult for patients to return for care. Shared decision-making can be used to help prioritize when and how the clinical preventive services are completed, and practices should have systems in place to facilitate patient follow-up as needed.

SUMMARY

Evidence-based clinical preventive services have the potential to reduce morbidity and mortality and optimize health. The passage of the ACA led to changes in policy that have increased coverage for several clinical preventive services, with no cost-sharing. The WPSI has worked to and continues to identify gaps in recommended preventive services for women. The Well-Woman Chart and the accompanying Clinical Summary Tables, which are updated annually and available online, can be used at the point of care to ensure women are offered and receive all the preventive services recommended for their age and circumstance. By using additional tools recommended through the Well-Woman Chart and the WPSI Web site, providers can more efficiently and effectively partner with their patients to optimize health and well-being.

DISCLAIMER

The opinions and assertions expressed herein are those of the author and do not reflect the official policy or position of the Uniformed Services University of the Health Sciences or the Department of Defense.

CLINICS CARE POINTS

- The WPSI Well-Woman Chart and Clinical Summary Tables provide a point-of-care resource for clinicians to determine which preventive services would be appropriate for a given patient.
- It may be impossible to complete all indicated clinical preventive services in one visit. Reassure the patient that they can be accomplished in a series of visits over time and ensure adequate follow-up is in place for the patient.
- Utlize shared decison-making to help prioritize when and how the clinical preventive services are completed.

DISCLOSURE

The author has nothing to disclose.

REFERENCES

1. Office of Disease Prevention and Health Promotion. Healthy People 2030. Healthcare Access and Quality. Available at: https://health.gov/healthypeople/objectives-and-data/browse-objectives/health-care-access-and-quality. Accessed March 20, 2023.
2. Borsky A, Zhan C, Miller T, et al. Few Americans receive all high-priority, appropriate clinical preventive services. Health Aff 2018;37(6):925-8.
3. Allen EM, Call KT, Beebe TJ, et al. Barriers to care and health care utilization among the publicly insured. Med Care 2017;55(3):207-14.
4. Stormo AR, Saraiya M, Hing E, et al. Women's clinical preventive services in the United States: who is doing what? JAMA Intern Med 2014;174(9):1512-4.
5. Kessler RC, Petukhova M, Sampson NA, et al. Twelve-month and lifetime prevalence and lifetime morbid risk of anxiety and mood disorders in the United States. Int J Methods Psychiatr Res 2012;21:169-84.
6. National Academies of Sciences. Engineering, and medicine; health and medicine division; board on population health and public health practice; committee on addressing evidence gaps in clinical prevention recommendations; clinical practice guidelines and the U.S. Preventive services task force. In: Lieu AT, Stratton K, Wojtowicz A, editors. Closing evidence gaps in clinical prevention. Washington (DC): National Academies Press (US); 2021. Available at: https://www.ncbi.nlm.nih.gov/books/NBK579835/. Accessed March 20, 2023.
7. U.S. Preventive Services Task Force. U.S. Preventive Services Task Force Procedure Manual. Rockville, MD; 2021. Available at: https://www.uspreventiveservicestaskforce.org/uspstf/about-uspstf/methods-and-processes/procedure-manual. Accessed March 20, 2023.
8. American Academy of Pediatrics. In: Hagan JF, Shaw JS, Duncan PM, editors. Bright futures: guidelines for health supervision of infants, children and adolescents. 4th edition. Elk Grove Village (IL): American Academy of Pediatrics; 2017.

9. American Academy of Pediatrics. Bright Futures. Available at: https://www.aap. org/en/practice-management/bright-futures. Accessed March 20, 2023.

10. Centers for Disease Control and Prevention. Advisory Committee on Immunization Practices (ACIP). Available at: https://www.cdc.gov/vaccines/acip/index. html. Accessed March 20, 2023.

11. Centers for Disease Control and Prevention. Advisory Committee on Immunization Practices (ACIP) Recommendations. Available at: https://www.cdc.gov/ vaccines/acip/recommendations.html. Accessed March 20, 2023.

12. Department of the Treasury, Internal Revenue Service. Coverage of certain preventive services under the Affordable Care Act. Final rules. Fed Regist 2015; 80:41317–47.

13. Institute of Medicine. Clinical preventive services for women: closing the gaps. Washington, DC: The National Academies Press; 2011.

14. Stolp H, Fox J. Increasing receipt of women's preventive services. J Women's Health (Larchmt) 2015;24(11):875–81.

15. Health Resources and Services Administration. Women's preventive services guidelines. Available at: https://www.hrsa.gov/womens-guidelines-2016/index. html. Accessed March 20, 2023.

16. Women's Preventive Services Initiative. Available at: https://www. womenspreventivehealth.org/. Accessed on April 20, 2023.

17. Women's Preventive Service Initiative. Methodology. Available at: https:// 149858107.v2.pressablecdn.com/wp-content/uploads/WPSI-Methodology-1.pdf. Accessed April 20, 2023.

18. Phipps MG, Son S, Zahn C, et al. Women's Preventive Services Initiative's Well-Woman Chart. Obstet Gynecol 2019;134(3):465–9.

19. Women's Preventive Services Initiative. Recommendations for well-woman care - a well-woman chart. Washington, DC: ACOG Foundation; 2023. Available at: https://149858107.v2.pressablecdn.com/wp-content/uploads/FINAL_WPSI_ WWC_11x17_2023.pdf. Accessed April 25, 2023.

20. Women's Preventive Services Initiative. Recommendations for well-woman care: clinical summary tables. Washington, DC: ACOG Foundation; 2023. Available at: https://149858107.v2.pressablecdn.com/wp-content/uploads/FINAL_WPSI_ ClinicalSummaryTables_2023.pdf. Accessed April 25, 2023.

21. Gregory KD, Chelmow D, Nelson HD, et al. Screening for anxiety in adolescent and adult women: a recommendation from the Women's Preventive Services Initiative. Ann Intern Med 2020;173:48–56.

22. Women's Preventive Services Initiative. Screening for Anxiety. 2020. Available at: https://www.womenspreventivehealth.org/recommendations/screening-for-anxiety/. Accessed April 20, 2023.

23. Nelson HD, Cantor A, Pappas M, et al. Screening for anxiety in adolescent and adult women: a systematic review for the women's preventive services initiative. Ann Intern Med 2020;173(1):29–41.

24. US Preventive Services Task Force. Screening for HIV infection: US preventive services task force recommendation statement. JAMA 2019;321(23): 2326–36.

25. Women's Preventive Services Initiative. Human Immunodeficiency Virus Preexposure Screening & Risk Assessment. 2020. Available at: https://www. womenspreventivehealth.org/recommendations/human-immunodeficiency-virus-infection/. Accessed April 20, 2023.

26. Bush K, Kivlahan DR, McDonell MB, et al. The AUDIT alcohol consumption questions (AUDIT-C): an effective brief screening test for problem drinking.

Ambulatory Care Quality Improvement Project (ACQUIP). Arch Intern Med 1998; 158:1789–95.

27. Sherin KM, Sinacore JM, Li XQ, et al. HITS: A short domestic violence screening tool for use in a family practice setting. Fam Med 1988;30(7):508–12.

28. Kroenke K, Spitzer RL, Williams W, et al. An ultra-brief screening scale for anxiety and depression: the PHQ-4. Psychosomatics 2009;50(6):613–21.

29. Löwe B, Wahl I, Rose M, et al. A 4-item measure of depression and anxiety: validation and standardization of the Patient Health Questionnaire-4 (PHQ-4) in the general population. J Affect Disord 2010;122(1–2):86–95.

30. O'Reilly N, Nelson HD, Conry JM, et al. Women's preventive services initiative. screening for urinary incontinence in women: a recommendation from the women's preventive services initiative. Ann Intern Med 2018 Sep 4;169(5):320–8.

31. Cardozo L, Staskin D, Currie B, et al. Validation of a bladder symptom screening tool in women with incontinence due to overactive bladder. Int Urogynecol J 2014;25:1655–63.

32. Women's Preventive Services Initiative. Coding Guide. Available at: https://www.womenspreventivehealth.org/wpsi-coding-guide/. Accessed April 7, 2023.

Addressing Obesity
Implementing Evidence-Based Lifestyle Prevention and Treatment Strategies in Clinical Practice

Peter T. Katzmarzyk, PhD

KEYWORDS

- Weight management • Primary care • Weight loss • Overweight

KEY POINTS

- Given the association between obesity and the subsequent development of numerous chronic conditions, the prevention and treatment of obesity has the potential to greatly improve health, especially in high-risk populations.
- Primary care and other clinical settings offer promising opportunities to address obesity and weight management.
- A large body of scientific evidence from pragmatic trials indicates that intensive lifestyle Interventions delivered in primary care settings can produce clinically significant weight loss.
- There is a need for more research using effectiveness-implementation designs to study the translation of evidence-based weight loss interventions into real-world settings.

BACKGROUND

Individuals who have obesity are at elevated risk for developing severe medical complications, such as cardiovascular disease, type 2 diabetes, and cancer.[1–3] Reducing body weight by as little as 3% to 5% results in meaningful health improvements in most patients, whereas weight loss exceeding 5% is associated with clinically significant outcomes including diabetes prevention, improvements in glycemic control, and improvements in cardiovascular risk factors such as high-density lipoprotein (HDL)-cholesterol and triglycerides.[4] In 2013, the American Medical Association recognized obesity as a disease state, which requires interventions for prevention and treatment.[5] This recognition opens the door for increased access to care and reduced stigma about the causes of obesity (ie, shifting the blame away from personal attributes).[6] Obesity used to be a relatively rare disease but has increased significantly in prevalence over the last several decades; in 1960, approximately 13% of adults had

Pennington Biomedical Research Center, 6400 Perkins Road, Baton Rouge, LA 70808, USA
E-mail address: Peter.Katzmarzyk@pbrc.edu

Med Clin N Am 107 (2023) 1025–1034
https://doi.org/10.1016/j.mcna.2023.06.011
0025-7125/23/© 2023 Elsevier Inc. All rights reserved.

obesity,[7] a proportion which climbed to 42% by 2017 to 2018 (**Fig. 1**).[8] Further, recent estimates indicate that the aggregate medical costs associated with obesity in the United States are upward of $261 billion annually.[9] Thus, obesity and its associated comorbidities are a major threat to public health in the United States.

Modern obesity prevention and treatment options offer a variety of choices for patients, including behavioral and lifestyle modification programs, pharmacotherapy for those at an increased risk of comorbidities, and metabolic/bariatric surgery for those with more extreme cases of obesity and cardiometabolic risk. The *2013 American Heart Association (AHA)/American College of Cardiology (ACC)/The Obesity Society (TOS) Guidelines for the Management of Overweight and Obesity in Adults* recommend that patients with overweight and obesity should participate in comprehensive lifestyle programs that assist in increasing physical activity and lowering dietary intake of calories through behavioral strategies.[10] The US Preventive Services Task Force also recommends physicians offer intensive behavioral interventions to individuals with a body mass index of 30 kg/m^2 or higher.[11] Metabolic/bariatric surgery options should be considered for patients with a body mass index (BMI) $\geq$ 40 kg/m^2 or BMI $\geq$35 kg/m^2 with obesity-related comorbidities and who have not responded to behavioral treatment.[10]

In 2018, there were an estimated 860 million office-based physician visits in the United States, and 51% of the visits occurred in primary care offices.[12] The main reason or primary diagnoses for 39% of office-based physician visits were to manage chronic diseases.[13] Therefore, primary care settings could be important for the prevention and treatment of obesity for large segments of the population. Primary care providers are trusted medical professionals and have a key role to play in the prevention and treatment of obesity. However, the sole reliance on primary care providers to deliver obesity treatment has limitations in part due to limited time available during office visits,[14] lack of training in behavioral therapy, and low reimbursement rates.[15–17] Focus groups also show that primary care providers endorse their patients' participation in weight loss programs, but they prefer a peripheral role.[18] Thus, it is important to investigate a variety of team-based collaborative care models to deliver weight loss treatment in primary care.

WHAT IS THE EVIDENCE?

A large body of evidence has accumulated on the role of primary care-based intensive lifestyle interventions for obesity treatment and management. **Fig. 2** presents

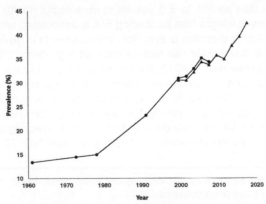

Fig. 1. Prevalence of adult obesity in the United States, 1960–1962 to 2017–2018. Results represented by closed circles are for adults 20 to 74 years of age (1960–1962 to 2007–2008),[7] and results represented by closed triangles are for adults 20+ years of age (1999–2000 to 2017–2018).[8]

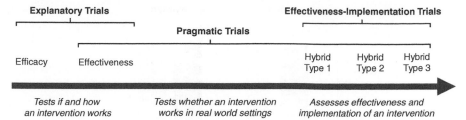

Fig. 2. Spectrum of human intervention trials. Human studies of weight loss range from carefully conducted explanatory trials to pragmatic trials that test effectiveness and implementation in real-world settings.

a schematic representation of the types of trials conducted in humans that have contributed evidence to this topic. Efficacy trials are studies aimed at testing whether an intervention (ie, exercise or dietary restriction) works to reduce obesity usually under ideal conditions; these trials are typically conducted under carefully controlled circumstances in laboratory settings. Effectiveness trials are also explanatory in nature and, depending on the design and setting, range in their level of pragmatism. Pragmatic trials *per se* are those conducted in real-world settings (schools, communities, health systems) and are designed to test if an intervention actually works when it is implemented in real-world human populations.[19] As you might expect, pragmatic trials range in their degree of pragmatism, and the PRECIS tool has been developed to help researchers assess the level of pragmatism in their trials.[20,21] Pragmatic trials may focus primarily on effectiveness, or they might also incorporate assessments of implementation, such as in effectiveness-implementation trials. Effectiveness-implementation trials typically will use one of three hybrid designs: hybrid type 1 trials test the effectiveness of an intervention while also gathering data on implementation; hybrid type 2 trials simultaneously test for clinical effectiveness and implementation strategies; and hybrid type 3 trials primarily test implementation strategies while gathering information about clinical effectiveness.[22] This article presents evidence on the role of intensive lifestyle interventions for obesity treatment and management across this spectrum of research studies.

Explanatory Trials

Several explanatory trials have established the efficacy and effectiveness of lifestyle-based obesity treatment and management strategies.[23–26] With respect to efficacy, carefully controlled laboratory studies have demonstrated that increasing energy expenditure through exercise or decreasing energy intake through dietary restriction promotes weight loss. **Fig. 3** presents the results of two carefully conducted laboratory efficacy trials: one conducted in men[27] and one conducted in women.[28] Over the course of several weeks, participants lost weight either by restricting dietary calories or increasing physical activity. Note that when the caloric deficit was carefully matched, similar weight loss was observed for diet and exercise. These studies demonstrate that weight loss is possible through dietary and exercise strategies under ideal laboratory conditions.

Pragmatic Trials

Seminal studies such as the Diabetes Prevention Program (DPP) and Action for Health in Diabetes (Look AHEAD) have established the effectiveness of intensive lifestyle interventions in achieving weight loss in community-dwelling humans.[29,30] After 4 years

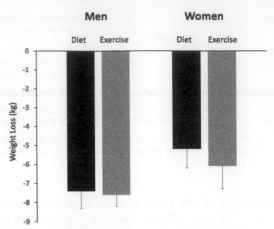

Fig. 3. Diet- and exercise-induced weight loss in men and women. Error bars represent one standard deviation. Men underwent 12 weeks of supervised intervention of ~700 kcal/day of dietary restriction or ~700 kcal/day of exercise energy expenditure.[27] Women underwent 14 weeks of supervised intervention of ~500 kcal/day of dietary restriction or ~500 kcal/day of exercise energy expenditure.[28]

of intervention, participants in the DPP intervention lost an average of 5.6 kg,[30] whereas those in the Look AHEAD intervention lost an average of 4.9 kg.[29] The DPP and Look AHEAD provide powerful evidence of the effectiveness of intensive lifestyle interventions at inducing clinically significant weight loss and positively impacting clinical outcomes for diabetes[30] and risk factors for cardiovascular disease.[31] However, these studies were conducted primarily in academic centers rather than in real-world settings such as physician offices or community health centers.

In 2006, the National Heart, Lung, and Blood Institute funded three pragmatic trials to test behavioral interventions for weight loss in primary care settings.[32] The POWER Hopkins trial was conducted in six primary care practices in Baltimore, Maryland.[33] A total of 415 patients with obesity and at least one cardiovascular risk factor were randomized to one of three groups: (1) control, (2) a remote support intervention delivered through the telephone, a study-specific Web site, and e-mail, or (3) an in-person support intervention which included group and individual sessions with a health coach in addition to telephone, a study-specific Web site, and e-mail support. After 2 years, the observed weight loss was 0.8, 4.6, and 5.1 kg in the control group, remote support, and in-person support groups, respectively.[33] The POWER-UP trial was conducted at the University of Pennsylvania in six primary care clinics owned by Penn Medicine.[34] A total of 380 adults with obesity were randomized to one of three groups: (1) usual care, (2) brief lifestyle counseling, or (3) or enhanced brief lifestyle intervention. After 2 years, the observed weight loss was 1.7, 2.9, and 4.6 kg for usual care, brief counseling, and the enhanced brief lifestyle intervention, respectively.[34] The Be Fit, Be Well trial was conducted in three community health centers in Boston, Massachusetts.[35] A total of 365 adults with obesity who were receiving hypertension treatment were randomized to one of two groups: (1) usual care or (2) a behavioral intervention that promoted weight loss and hypertension self-management using eHealth components. After 2 years, the observed weight loss was 0.5 and 1.5 kg for the usual care and behavioral intervention groups, respectively.[35]

In 2015, the Patient-Centered Outcomes Research Institute funded two large pragmatic trials to study obesity treatment options in underserved primary care settings.[36,37] The *RE-POWER* trial was conducted at the University of Kansas Medical Center in 36 primary care practices in the Midwestern United States.[38] A total of 1432 patients with obesity were randomized to one of three groups: (1) in-clinic individual visits, (2) in-clinic group visits, or (3) telephone group visits. After 2 years, the observed weight loss was 2.6, 4.4, and 3.9 kg in the in-clinic individual intervention, in-clinic group intervention, and the telephone group intervention, respectively.[38] The *PROPEL* trial was conducted by the Pennington Biomedical Research Center in Baton Rouge, Louisiana, in 18 primary care clinics primarily serving low-income patients.[39] A total of 803 patients with obesity were randomized to one of two groups: (1) usual care or (2) an in-clinic intensive lifestyle intervention. After 2 years, the observed weight loss was 0.9 and 5.4 kg in the usual care and intensive lifestyle intervention groups, respectively.[39]

Fig. 4 presents the mean weight loss across all treatment arms in the *POWER Hopkins, POWER-UP, Be Fit, Be Well, RE-POWER,* and *PROPEL* trials at 2 years. The weight loss observed in the usual care or control groups is less than 1 to 2 kg on average. On the other hand, several of the lifestyle interventions achieved clinically significant weight loss in the range of 3 to 5 kg. Although all the trials were pragmatic, the degree of pragmatism varied across trials and study arms. Therefore, careful consideration should be given to selecting and implementing these evidence-based strategies based on the health care setting and resources available to support the intervention.

Systematic Reviews

The previous sections have provided a summary of carefully conducted weight loss trials conducted in a variety of settings and populations. These studies have contributed to a larger body of evidence on weight loss efforts in clinical settings. Several narrative and systematic reviews have tackled this issue over the years, and most recently, two systematic reviews have summarized the published research on this topic. The first review summarized data from 56 articles published between 2000

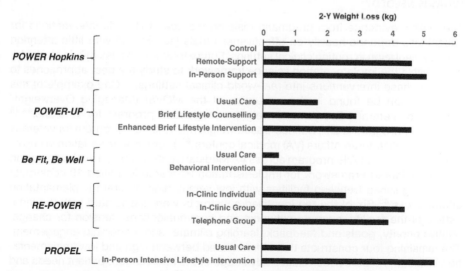

Fig. 4. Mean weight loss across treatment arms in several pragmatic trials of obesity treatment and management in primary care settings. The trials included POWER Hopkins,[33] POWER-UP,[34] Be Fit, Be Well,[35] REPOWER,[38] and PROPEL.[39]

and 2020, representing 72 interventions.[40] Although the investigators did not conduct a formal meta-analysis, they concluded that "most" interventions were effective at reducing BMI, body weight, and waist circumference. Among 67 interventions where body weight was an outcome, 37 produced a significant effect.[40] The investigators also noted that most of the studies were conducted in high-income countries, and there is a need for more research in low- and middle-income countries. The second review conducted a meta-analysis and summarized data from 34 trials (mostly from high-income countries).[41] The results indicated a mean difference between intervention and comparator groups of −2.3 kg (95% confidence interval = −3.0 to −1.6 kg) for weight loss at 12 months and a mean difference of −1.8 kg (95% confidence interval = −2.8 to −0.8 kg) at 24 months favoring the intervention groups.[41]

WHAT DO THE GUIDELINES SAY?

A recent systematic review summarized international evidence-based guidelines for the management of overweight and obesity.[42] A total of 19 guidelines published between 2012 and 2018 were identified; 10 were from the United States, 3 from the United Kingdom, 2 from Germany, and 1 each from Canada, Australia, Spain, and a European medical society. All but three of the guidelines included recommendations for lifestyle changes including diet and physical activity. In general, the guidelines recommend the use of comprehensive lifestyle interventions of at least 6 to 12 months in duration, focusing on reducing calories, increasing physical activity, and incorporating measures to support behavioral change.[42]

From the North American perspective, the most comprehensive guidelines for adults are the *2013 AHA/ACC/TOS Guidelines for the Management of Overweight and Obesity in Adults*[10] in the United States and the *Canadian Adult Obesity Clinical Practice Guidelines*.[43] Both of these guidelines recommend multicomponent behavioral interventions for adults with obesity. **Box 1** presents the specific recommendations from these guidelines that relate to multicomponent weight loss interventions.

WHAT IS NEEDED?

The current evidence from pragmatic trials on the use of lifestyle interventions for weight loss depends heavily on effectiveness trials (see **Fig. 2**) with little attention to implementation in routine clinical settings. Future trials should use hybrid study designs within the implementation science framework to study the best approaches to translate these interventions into real-world clinical settings.[22] One example of this approach can be found in the evaluation of the *MOVE!* (Managing Overweight/Obesity for Veterans Everywhere) weight management program for veterans.[44,45] The *MOVE!* program is an evidence-based weight management program for veterans available in all Veteran Affairs (VA) medical centers.[44] There is wide variation in implementation of the MOVE! program across VA Medical Centers, and an evaluation using the Consolidated Framework for Implementation Research identified 10 constructs that distinguished between facilities with low versus high program implementation effectiveness.[45] Six of the ten identified constructs were associated with the inner setting of the facility, such as networks and communications, tension for change, relative priority, goals and feedback, learning climate, and leadership engagement. The remaining four constructs that differentiated between high and low implementation included the perceived relative advantage of the intervention, patient needs and resources, executing, and reflecting and evaluating.[45] The results and recommendations generated by this research can be used to improve program implementation across all sites, and the results suggest that characteristics of the inner settings

> **Box 1**
> **Specific recommendations relating to multicomponent weight loss interventions from selected current obesity prevention and treatment guidelines relating to multicomponent weight loss interventions**
>
> 2013 AHA/ACC/TOS Guidelines for the Management of Overweight and Obesity in Adults[10]
> - Advise overweight and obese individuals who would benefit from weight loss to participate for ≥6 months in a comprehensive lifestyle program that assists participants in adhering to a lower calorie diet and in increasing physical activity through the use of behavioral strategies.
> - Prescribe on-site, high-intensity (ie, ≥14 sessions in 6 months) comprehensive weight loss interventions provided in individual or group sessions by a trained interventionist.
>
> Canadian Adult Obesity Clinical Practice Guidelines[43]
> - Multicomponent psychological interventions (combining behavior modification [goal-setting, self-monitoring, problem-solving], cognitive therapy [reframing], and value-based strategies to alter diet and activity) should be incorporated into care plans for weight loss and improved health status and quality of life in a manner that promotes adherence, confidence, and intrinsic motivation.
> - Primary care multicomponent programs should consider personalized obesity management strategies as an effective way to support people living with obesity.
> - Primary care interventions that are behavior-based (nutrition, exercise, lifestyle), alone or in combination with pharmacotherapy, should be used to manage overweight and obesity.
> - Group-based diet and physical activity sessions informed by the Diabetes Prevention Program and the Look AHEAD (Action for Health in Diabetes) programs should be used as an effective management option for adults with overweight and obesity.

(facilities in this case) may be important constructs to pay attention to early in the intervention planning process.

SUMMARY

Obesity treatment and management has progressed from a strong evidence-base of explanatory trials providing data that dietary restriction increases in physical activity, and behavioral strategies are effective at achieving weight loss in humans. Over the last decade, several pragmatic trials conducted in routine clinical settings have demonstrated that clinically significant weight loss is possible with multicomponent intensive lifestyle intervention. The observed weight losses in these trials are consistent with the prevention of several chronic diseases and alterations in disease progression trajectories. Further research is required to study the best way to implement these strategies in different clinical settings using implementation science study designs.

CLINICS CARE POINTS

> - Multicomponent lifestyle interventions with a focus on weight loss are effective strategies to prevent chronic disease and slow chronic disease progression in adults.
> - Primary care clinics represent an underused environment for the treatment and management of obesity.
> - Patients with obesity should be referred to multicomponent comprehensive weight loss interventions.
> - When choosing which evidence-based program to implement, careful consideration should be given to the balance between effectiveness, pragmatism, and resources available to conduct the intervention.

• Primary care clinicians should participate in future research on weight loss to improve the health of their patients and future generations of patients.

DISCLOSURE

The author has nothing to disclose.

FUNDING

This work was funded, in part, by the Patient-Centered Outcomes Research Institute (Award OB-1402-10977), grant U54 GM104940 from the National Institute of General Medical Sciences of the National Institutes of Health (NIH), which funds the Louisiana Clinical and Translational Science Center, and by grant P30DK072476 from the National Institute of Diabetes and Digestive and Kidney Diseases of NIH which funds the Pennington/Louisiana Nutrition Obesity Research Center.

REFERENCES

1. Guh DP, Zhang W, Bansback N, et al. The incidence of co-morbidities related to obesity and overweight: a systematic review and meta-analysis. BMC Public Health 2009;9:88.
2. Lauby-Secretan B, Scoccianti C, Loomis D, et al. Body fatness and cancer–viewpoint of the IARC working group. N Engl J Med 2016;375(8):794–8.
3. Poirier P, Giles TD, Bray GA, et al. Obesity and cardiovascular disease: pathophysiology, evaluation, and effect of weight loss: an update of the 1997 American heart association scientific statement on obesity and heart disease from the obesity committee of the council on nutrition, physical activity, and metabolism. Circulation 2006;113(6):898–918.
4. Ryan DH, Yockey SR. Weight loss and improvement in comorbidity: differences at 5%, 10%, 15%, and over. Curr Obes Rep 2017;6(2):187–94.
5. Pollack A. AMA recognizes obesity as a disease. NYTimescom. Available at: https://www.nytimes.com/2013/06/19/business/ama-recognizes-obesity-as-a-disease.html.
6. Kyle TK, Dhurandhar EJ, Allison DB. Regarding obesity as a disease: evolving policies and their implications. Endocrinol Metab Clin North Am 2016;45(3):511–20.
7. Ogden CL, Carroll MD. Prevalence of overweight, obesity, and extreme obesity among adults: United States, trends 1960–1962 through 2007–2008. NCHS Health E-Stat; Available at: https://www.cdc.gov/nchs/data/hestat/obesity_adult_07_08/obesity_adult_07_08.pdf. June 2010.
8. Hales CM, Carroll MD, Fryar CD, et al. Prevalence of obesity and severe obesity among adults: United States, 2017-2018. NCHS Data Brief 2020;(360):1–8.
9. Cawley J, Biener A, Meyerhoefer C, et al. Direct medical costs of obesity in the United States and the most populous states. J Manag Care Spec Pharm 2021;27(3):354–66.
10. Jensen MD, Ryan DH, Apovian CM, et al. 2013 AHA/ACC/TOS guideline for the management of overweight and obesity in adults: a report of the American college of cardiology/American heart association task force on practice guidelines and the obesity society. Circulation 2014;129(25 Suppl.2):S102–38.
11. U.S. Preventive Services Task Force. Screening for and management of obesity in adults: U.S. Preventive services task force recommendation statement. Ann Intern Med 2012;157:373–8.

12. Santo L, Okeyode T. National Ambulatory Medical Care Survey: 2018 National Summary Tables. Available at: https://www.cdc.gov/nchs/data/ahcd/namcs_summary/2018-namcs-web-tables-508.pdf.

13. Ashman JJ, Santo L, Okeyode T. Characteristics of office-based physician visits, 2018. NCHS data brief, no. 408. Hyattsville, MD: National Center for Health Statistics; 2021. p. 7.

14. Kaplan LM, Golden A, Jinnett K, et al. Perceptions of barriers to effective obesity care: results from the national ACTION study. Obesity 2018;26(1):61–9.

15. Carvajal R, Wadden TA, Tsai AG, et al. Managing obesity in primary care practice: a narrative review. Ann NY Acad Sci 2013;1281:191–206.

16. Pagoto SL, Pbert L, Emmons K, et al. Society of behavioral medicine public policy leadership group. policy brief: the society for behavioral medicine position statement on the CMS decision memo on intensive behavioral therapy for obesity. Transl Behav Med 2012;2(4):381–3.

17. Smith S, Seeholzer EL, Gullett H, et al. Primary care residents' knowledge, attitudes, self-efficacy, and perceived professional norms regarding obesity, nutrition, and physical activity counseling. J Grad Med Educ 2015;7:388–94.

18. Bennett WL, Gudzune KA, Appel LJ, et al. Insights from the POWER practice-based weight loss trial: a focus group study on the PCP's role in weight management. J Gen Intern Med 2014;29(1):50–8.

19. Patsopoulos NA. A pragmatic view on pragmatic trials. Dialogues Clin Neurosci 2011;13(2):217–24.

20. Loudon K, Treweek S, Sullivan F, et al. The PRECIS 2 tool: designing trials that are fit for purpose. BMJ 2015;350:h2147.

21. Thorpe KE, Zwarenstein M, Oxman AD, et al. A pragmatic-explanatory continuum indicator summary (PRECIS): a tool to help trial designers. J Clin Epidemiol 2009; 62(5):464–75.

22. Curran GM, Bauer M, Mittman B, et al. Effectiveness-implementation hybrid designs: combining elements of clinical effectiveness and implementation research to enhance public health impact. Med Care 2012;50(3):217–26.

23. Donnelly JE, Blair SN, Jakicic JM, et al. American college of sports medicine position stand. appropriate physical activity intervention strategies for weight loss and prevention of weight regain for adults. Med Sci Sports Exerc 2009;41(2):459–71.

24. Jakicic JM, Powell KE, Campbell WW, et al. Physical activity and the prevention of weight gain in adults: a systematic review. Med Sci Sports Exerc 2019;51(6):1262–9.

25. Raynor HA, Champagne CM. Position of the academy of nutrition and dietetics: interventions for the treatment of overweight and obesity in adults. J Acad Nutr Diet 2016;116(1):129–47.

26. Brown J, Clarke C, Johnson Stoklossa C, Sievenpiper J. Canadian adult obesity clinical practice guidelines: medical nutrition therapy in obesity management. Available at: https://obesitycanadaca/guidelines/nutrition. Accessed January 27, 2023 2022.

27. Ross R, Dagnone D, Jones PJ, et al. Reduction in obesity and related comorbid conditions after diet-induced weight loss or exercise-induced weight loss in men. A randomized, controlled trial. Ann Intern Med 2000;133(2):92–103.

28. Ross R, Janssen I, Dawson J, et al. Exercise-induced reduction in obesity and insulin resistance in women: a randomized controlled trial. Obes Res 2004;12:789–98.

29. Look Ahead Research Group, Wing RR. Long-term effects of a lifestyle intervention on weight and cardiovascular risk factors in individuals with type 2 diabetes mellitus: four-year results of the Look AHEAD trial. Arch Intern Med 2010;170(17): 1566–75.

30. Diabetes Prevention Program Research Group. Reduction in the incidence of type 2 diabetes with lifestyle intervention or metformin. N Engl J Med 2002;346: 393–403.

31. Wing RR, Lang W, Wadden TA, et al. Benefits of modest weight loss in improving cardiovascular risk factors in overweight and obese individuals with type 2 diabetes. Diabetes Care 2011;34(7):1481–6.

32. Yeh HC, Clark JM, Emmons KE, et al. Independent but coordinated trials: insights from the practice-based opportunities for weight reduction trials collaborative research group. Clin Trials 2010;7(4):322–32.

33. Appel LJ, Clark JM, Yeh HC, et al. Comparative effectiveness of weight-loss interventions in clinical practice. N Engl J Med 2011;365(21):1959–68.

34. Wadden TA, Volger S, Sarwer DB, et al. A two-year randomized trial of obesity treatment in primary care practice. N Engl J Med 2011;365(21):1969–79.

35. Bennett GG, Warner ET, Glasgow RE, et al. Obesity treatment for socioeconomically disadvantaged patients in primary care practice. Arch Intern Med 2012; 172(7):565–74.

36. Katzmarzyk PT, Martin CK, Newton RL Jr, et al. Promoting successful weight loss in primary care in louisiana (PROPEL): rationale, design and baseline characteristics. Contemp Clin Trials 2018;67:1–10.

37. Befort CA, VanWormer JJ, DeSouza C, et al. Protocol for the rural engagement in primary care for optimizing weight reduction (RE-POWER) trial: comparing three obesity treatment models in rural primary care. Contemp Clin Trials 2016;47: 304–14.

38. Befort CA, VanWormer JJ, Desouza C, et al. Effect of behavioral therapy with in-clinic or telephone group visits vs in-clinic individual visits on weight loss among patients with obesity in rural clinical practice: a randomized clinical trial. JAMA 2021;325(4):363–72.

39. Katzmarzyk PT, Martin CK, Newton RL Jr, et al. Weight loss in underserved patients - A cluster-randomized trial. N Engl J Med 2020;383(10):909–18.

40. Marques ES, Interlenghi GS, Leite TH, et al. Primary care-based interventions for treatment of obesity: a systematic review. Public Health 2021;195:61–9.

41. Madigan CD, Graham HE, Sturgiss E, et al. Effectiveness of weight management interventions for adults delivered in primary care: systematic review and meta-analysis of randomised controlled trials. BMJ 2022;377:e069719.

42. Semlitsch T, Stigler FL, Jeitler K, et al. Management of overweight and obesity in primary care-A systematic overview of international evidence-based guidelines. Obes Rev 2019;20(9):1218–30.

43. Wharton S, Lau DCW, Vallis M, et al. Obesity in adults: a clinical practice guideline. CMAJ (Can Med Assoc J) 2020;192(31):E875–91.

44. Kinsinger LS, Jones KR, Kahwati L, et al. Design and dissemination of the MOVE! weight-management program for veterans. Prev Chronic Dis 2009;6(3):A98.

45. Damschroder LJ, Lowery JC. Evaluation of a large-scale weight management program using the consolidated framework for implementation research (CFIR). Implement Sci 2013;8:51.

Treatment Updates for Pain Management and Opioid Use Disorder

Thomas Locke, MD, MPH[a,*], Elizabeth Salisbury-Afshar, MD, MPH[b], David Tyler Coyle, MD, MS[a]

KEYWORDS

- Opioids • Pain • Opioid use disorder • Contingency management
- Stimulant use disorder • Naloxone

KEY POINTS

- Non-opioid therapies are at least as effective as opioids for many common types of acute pain.
- Substance Abuse and Mental Health Services Administration's pandemic era flexibility with take-home methadone doses from Opioid Treatment Programs has continued after being met with strong support from both patients and providers.
- Low-dose initiation of buprenorphine can be an effective approach to treating patients with opioid use disorder. Patients do *not* need to enter withdrawal for a low-dose buprenorphine initiation.
- Concomitant opioid and stimulant use is on the increase, as are fatal overdoses involving polysubstance use. Contingency management—the practice of incentivizing patients for abstinence from drug use—has a demonstrated track record of decreasing stimulant use while increasing treatment engagement across a variety of care settings.
- Naloxone can be dispensed from pharmacies without a prescription in all states via standing order. Over-the-counter naloxone products were recently approved by the US FDA and are expected to be available in the second half of 2023.

INTRODUCTION

The number of Americans with opioid use disorder (OUD) has steadily risen over the past 2 decades, now affecting roughly 2.7 million adults.[1] The number of drug overdose deaths has risen dramatically in the past 5 years. Nearly 107,000 people died of drug overdose in the 12 months ending in April 2021, representing a nearly fivefold rate increase (32.4 vs 6.8 per 100,000 standard population) compared with 2001.

[a] University of Colorado School of Medicine, 13001 East 17th Place, Aurora, CO 80045, USA; [b] University of Wisconsin School of Medicine and Public Health, 610 North Whitney Way, Suite 200, Madison, WI 53705, USA
* Corresponding author.
E-mail address: Thomas.locke@cuanschutz.edu

Med Clin N Am 107 (2023) 1035–1046
https://doi.org/10.1016/j.mcna.2023.06.017
medical.theclinics.com

Synthetic opioids, including fentanyl, are driving mortality[2] Evidence-based interventions are essential to combat the extraordinary challenges associated with opioid use in high-risk populations; the authors aim to review this evidence to support clinical decision-making in primary care practices.

Updates to Chronic Pain Management with Opioids

In March 2016, the US Centers for Disease Control and Prevention (CDC) published their "Guidelines for Prescribing Opioids for Chronic Pain" for primary care physicians (PCPs).[3] These guidelines were created to help PCPs decide whether to initiate and/or continue opioids for patients with chronic pain, guide opioid selection, and inform dosage recommendations. The guideline used a 4-tiered evidence-type scale based on the Agency for Healthcare Research and Quality's (AHRQ) adaptation of the Advisory Committee on Immunization Practices (ACIP) Grading of Recommendation, Assessment, Development and Evaluation method (**Table 1**).[3]

Of the 12 recommendations in the 2016 Guidelines, none cited Type 1 evidence and only one cited Type 2 evidence. Seven recommendations cited Type 4 evidence. Type 4 evidence is equivalent to AHRQs "low strength of evidence with serious limitations" with the ACIPs Type 4 evidence indicating "very little confidence in the effect estimate (high uncertainty), and the likelihood is high that the true effect differs from the estimate of the effect." The 2016 guidelines also provided specific milligram morphine equivalent (MME) recommendations to avoid exceeding based largely on expert opinion. This is notable as there is no evidence that there exists a threshold MME beyond which risk increases; rather, risk increases as dose increases.[4]

Six years later, the updated 2022 CDC Clinical Practice Guideline for Prescribing Opioids for Pain continues to rely on low-quality evidence.[5] Only one recommendation draws from Type 1 evidence, one with Type 2 evidence, and seven based on Type 4 evidence. Specific MME recommendations have been removed. The updated guidelines include "acute" and "subacute" pain in several of their recommendations. The updated guidelines also offer recommendations for patients who are already receiving opioid therapy and how physicians can discuss the risks and benefits around medication tapering. The updated guidelines also attempt to address health equity with a paragraph outlining the inequalities in the introduction and a brief mention of the concept in the conclusion. However, no recommendations explicitly mention healthy equity. The omission from the recommendations means many who read solely the recommendation bullet points may miss this content. Including equity content—even those based on low-quality evidence—may valuably add to future revisions of the recommendations.

Table 1
Centers for Disease Control and Prevention opioid prescribing guideline tiers of evidence quality

Evidence Quality	Type	Description
Strongest	1	Randomized clinical trials or overwhelming evidence from observational studies.
	2	Randomized clinical trials with important limitations or exceptionally strong evidence from observational studies.
	3	Observational studies or randomized clinical trials with notable limitations.
Weakest	4	Clinical experience and observations, observational studies with important limitations, or randomized clinical trials with several major limitations.

Two recommendations in the 2022 Practice Guideline are based on strong data support. The recommendations advising providers to start with non-opioid analgesic agents before moving to opioids (#2, Type 2 evidence) and to refer patients with OUD to evidence-based treatment (#12, Type 1 evidence) have a more rigorous evidence base than the other guidelines. Both recommendations improved their evidence grade from the previous guidelines. This improvement is encouraging and highlights the potential for other recommendations to similarly develop in future iterations of the guidelines. Indeed, the CDC guidelines read: "Although the strength of the evidence is sometimes low quality and research gaps remain, clinical scientific evidence continues to advance and supports the recommendations in this clinical practice guideline." A major challenge in studying the use of opioids for pain is that not all types of pain are the same, and the subjective experience of pain makes it difficult to quantify.

CLINICS CARE POINTS

- Updates to Guidelines:
  - Acute pain (duration <1 month): Non-opioid therapies are at least as effective as opioids for many common types of acute pain.
  - Subacute pain (duration 1–3 months): Non-opioid therapies are preferred for subacute and chronic pain (duration >3 months).
  - Many noninvasive non-pharmacologic approaches, including physical and behavioral therapy, can improve pain and function with very low risk.
  - Clinicians, practices, health systems, and payers should be mindful of health equity and implicit bias in managing the pain of all kinds of patients.
  - For patients already receiving opioid therapy:
    - Be careful when changing opioid dosage and avoid rapid dose decreases.
    - Opioid therapy should not be discontinued abruptly.
    - Use the lowest effective opioid dose in treating pain whenever opioids are indicated and maximize concomitant non-opioid therapy.

Updates to Opioid Use Disorder Treatment in Primary Care Settings

The early stages of the COVID-19 pandemic presented several challenges for Opioid Treatment Programs (OTPs). OTPs, federally licensed clinics that dispense methadone, are required to offer in-person care. Pre-pandemic patients who began treatment at an OTP were required by federal regulation to attend the clinic in-person 6 days per week for the first several months of treatment, with the possibility of receiving take-home doses slowly increasing thereafter. The prospect of mandating in-person clinic attendance daily during an era of social distancing proved sufficiently concerning for regulators to change this requirement. In March 2020, the Substance Abuse and Mental Health Services Administration (SAMHSA) issued an exemption allowing states to request that their OTPs can provide up to 28 days of take-home doses of methadone for patients meeting certain criteria.[6] Three years later, states, OTPs, and patients continue to support this exemption. Advocates identify an increase in treatment engagement, improved patient satisfaction, and fewer incidents of misuse associated with greater methadone take-home flexibility.[7,8] The exemption remains in place today, and SAMHSA has indicated that it may become permanent; however, a final decision has yet to be announced.[9]

On the coattails of the successful changes around methadone dispensed from OTPs, advocates have called for reform to the methadone regulatory framework. The National Institute on Drug Abuse convened a Methadone Access Research Task Force to develop a research agenda to increase access to methadone treatment for OUD. One prong of this agenda includes exploring the risks and benefits of expanded methadone access in the United States.[10] The support of a federal agency in exploring this topic is significant, suggesting an openness to reforming a system largely unchanged since the 1970s.

The pandemic also improved access to substance use disorder care by increasing availability and awareness of telemedicine. Telemedicine offers safe, accessible health care and delivers outcomes similar to "care as usual" for OUD.[11,12] One study found patients with Medicare had increased retention in care and a reduced odds of medically treated overdose when receiving medication management for OUD via tele-health services.[12] Another study found video observation of methadone take-home doses as an effective alternative to in-person dosing.[13]

Although telemedicine has certainly increased access to care, the reintroduction of mobile treatment units has brought medicine straight to the people. Many persons seeking treatment for OUD must travel long distances to receive methadone at a brick-and-mortar OTP, with longer travel distances associated with worse treatment outcomes.[14] To address this disparity, the drug enforcement administration (DEA) allowed mobile methadone units to provide legally dispensed methadone to people in need at specified parking locations. For 2 decades, mobile methadone mobile units provided care. From 2007 to 2021, the approval of new units was paused by the DEA and ultimately resumed in July 2021.[15] DEA-registered OTPs may once again obtain and deploy mobile methadone units, with the goal of increasing access to care in underserved areas.

Another recent policy change was the elimination of the DATA-Waiver through the Consolidated Appropriations Act of 2023—which includes elements of Mainstreaming of Addiction Treatment Act and the Medication Access and Training Expansion Act.[16] The DATA-Waiver (also called the X-Waiver) required additional training for DEA-licensed providers—8 hours for physicians, 24 hours for advanced practice providers—as well as administrative burden and patient limits to prescribe buprenorphine for OUD. With the X-Waiver removal, providers with a DEA registration with Schedule III authority can prescribe buprenorphine to patients with OUD without any limitations, including no limitations on the number of patients treated. The DEA and SAMHSA plan to implement new training requirements for all DEA-licensed prescribers, which are expected to go into effect in June 2023.[17]

Another update related to OUD treatment involves a novel change in clinical practice in response to the increasing concentration of fentanyl in the non-pharmaceutical opioid supply. Low-dose initiation of buprenorphine is a relatively new approach for transitioning patients from full opioid agonists to buprenorphine. Buprenorphine, a partial mu-opioid agonist with high affinity for the receptor, can cause precipitated withdrawal (PW) if a full dose is administered to a patient who has recently used full agonist opioids. In a traditional buprenorphine initiation, patients using full agonist opioids must abstain from opioid use until entering mild-to-moderate withdrawal—an unappetizing prospect for many patients—then begin buprenorphine slowly. The emergence of widespread illicit fentanyl use, and fentanyl's high lipophilicity, has led to increased concerns related to traditional initiations causing more PW. This phenomenon is not universal, with data on the incidence of PW related to buprenorphine initiation somewhat limited: ED-based studies have shown an incidence of ~1%, and other data based on patient self-reported data have shown an incidence of 35% to 40% depending on a variety of factors.[18,19] In response, prescribers have embraced low-dose buprenorphine initiation. Multiple studies have demonstrated its effectiveness and tolerability.[20] The process begins with a small dose of buprenorphine and increasing dose gradually, all while the patient continues to use the full agonist opioids (**Table 2**).

Table 2
Example schedule for low dose initiation of buprenorphine

Day	Buprenorphine Dose	Continue Other Opioid?
1	0.5 mg once a day	Yes
2	0.5 mg twice a day	Yes
3	1 mg twice a day	Yes
4	2 mg twice a day	Yes
5	3 mg twice a day	Yes
6	4 mg twice a day	Yes
7	4 mg thrice a day (stop other opioids)	No
8	12–20 mg total daily dose	No

During this time, the patient continues to use full agonist opioids.[20] On reaching 12 mg, the patient is instructed to stop their full agonist opioid and is given a full dose of buprenorphine (typically 12–24 mg) aiming to avoid PW and successfully transitioning to buprenorphine. This approach has been studied most extensively in the inpatient setting; however, positive data exist from the ambulatory setting as well.

CLINICS CARE POINTS

- SAMHSAs pandemic era flexibility with take-home methadone doses from OTPs has continued after being met with strong support from OTPs and patients.
- Telemedicine and mobile methadone units are two proven strategies to improve access to OUD treatment.
- The X Waiver has been eliminated; providers are able to prescribe buprenorphine for OUD with a standard DEA registration.
- Low-dose initiation of buprenorphine can be an effective approach to treating patients with OUD, particularly if there is concern about PW or inability to tolerate withdrawal. Patients do *not* need to enter withdrawal for a low-dose buprenorphine initiation.

Concomitant Stimulant and Opioid Use and Increased Access to Contingency Management

Concomitant stimulant and opioid use continues to increase in the United States with some researchers deeming our current era the "fourth wave" of the opioid epidemic.[21–23] At present, there are no FDA-approved medications to treat methamphetamine or cocaine use disorders.[24] Providers must rely on psychosocial treatments to treat patients with stimulant use disorders, and the behavioral intervention with the strongest evidence base to treat stimulant use disorders is contingency management.

Contingency management (CM) is a psychosocial intervention where participants are rewarded for positive behavior.[25] In relation to stimulant use disorders, CM is used to incentivize abstinence from drug use. In practice, patients who provide a negative toxicology test are rewarded, and this reward builds on itself with repeated negative toxicology tests over time. Rewards may be a coupon, gift card, or a cash prize.

Critics argue CM is a poor use of limited resources, stating it is unethical to pay people for what they "should be doing anyway."[26] However, CM is both clinically effective and cost beneficial. A recent systematic review examined the practice of CM among patients with methamphetamine use disorder, finding the intervention not only decreased non-prescribed substance use but also lower rates of medical utilization and risky sexual behaviors.[27] Other studies of methamphetamine and cocaine use disorders have supported this evidence with similar results: CM is consistently associated with improved clinical outcomes and is more effective than other behavioral interventions.[28,29] An economic analysis of stimulant use disorder treatments in a community setting found CM was an overall cost saving intervention when used in conjunction with other psychosocial interventions, such as cognitive behavioral therapy.[29]

Despite its efficacy, CM has not been widely adopted by providers and treatment centers. One reason for this low uptake is the lack of a mechanism for reimbursement. However, state Medicaid programs have leveraged Section 1115 of the Social Security Act to request waivers creating pilot programs that increase availability of CM by using Medicaid funding.[30] Montana and California Medicaid plans now offer a CM benefit.[31,32] The California program—named the Recovery Incentives Program—began in the first quarter of 2023 for eligible California Medicaid beneficiaries. It is expected to run for 24 weeks with an upgraded incentive change in the latter 12 weeks pending patient participation.[32] Although models may vary across states, the California program caps the yearly reimbursement at $599 per patient.[33] Other states, including Washington and West Virginia, are also piloting CM programs.[34,35]

CLINICS CARE POINTS

- Concomitant opioid and stimulant use is on the rise, as are fatal overdoses involving polysubstance use.
- There are no FDA-approved medications for cocaine or methamphetamine use disorders.
- CM—the practice of incentivizing patients for abstinence from drug use—has a demonstrated track record of decreasing stimulant use while increasing treatment engagement across a variety of care settings.
- CM will likely continue to be implemented in the future as more payors offer reimbursement.

Updates on Naloxone Access

Naloxone, an opioid receptor antagonist used as an antidote to opioid overdoses, is an essential tool in the medical management of OUD. Policymakers, pharmacists, patients, and providers all support increasing access to naloxone; however, the optimal path to this outcome is debated. Removing the requirement for an individual prescription has proven effective: Ohio's dispensed naloxone orders increased by 2328% over a 3 year time period following the removal of this requirement.[36] Other studies have found similar increases in Medicaid recipient dispensing following similar changes.[37] Currently, pharmacists in all 50 states can dispense naloxone without a patient-specific prescription through the use of statewide standing orders.[38] Pharmacy access may be particularly important for communities that do not have local harm reduction programs.

Although this policy change has allowed greater access to naloxone, medication cost remains a barrier to widespread distribution. The drugmaker Kaleo famously raised the cost of its naloxone auto-injector Evzio by 600% to $4100 per dose; the drugmaker later entered into a $12.7 million settlement with the Department of Justice to resolve allegations of false claims related to falsified prior authorizations related to its extraordinary price hike.[39,40] The overwhelming majority of naloxone dispensed in the United States is as a nasal spray. The out-of-pocket cost for naloxone can range from $60 to $140 (for one box containing two doses).[41–43] With Medicaid, generic naloxone averages around $20 with state-to-state variability.[43] Price is not the only barrier; 10 states have monthly prescription limits, seven having top-10 per-capita opioid prescribing rates nationwide.[44]

Of note, a federal advisory committee recommended the US Food and Drug Administration authorize over-the-counter naloxone in February 2023, paving the way for even greater access to the drug.[45] Many states also have third party prescribing, which allows someone to receive naloxone with the intention of using the product on someone else.[46] In addition to government efforts, nonprofit organizations have developed resources aiming to link providers and patients with freely dispensed naloxone nationwide.[47,48] Medication cost is particularly important for nonprofit organizations focusing on harm reduction: the cheaper the product, the more units that can be purchased and distributed to high-need populations.

Providers and organizations are striving to increase naloxone access in ambulatory and emergency department settings. Co-prescription of naloxone with opioids has increased over the past decade.[49] The 2016 CDC Guideline for Prescribing Opioids for Chronic Pain recommended providers consider co-prescribing naloxone to patients taking greater than 50 MME opioids per day; however, the updated 2022 guidelines offer no specific recommendations for MME dosages above which naloxone co-prescribing should occur, instead leaving the decision to the judgment of the provider.[3,5] Naloxone co-prescribing has increased across all states, but individual state rates vary and co-prescribed naloxone rates nationally are low overall.[50–51] Importantly, evidence supporting co-prescription as an effective means to reduce opioid overdose on a population level is limited.[51] Nevertheless, given potential benefit and limited risk, greater distribution of naloxone among people who need it is a promising approach.

Naloxone prescriptions are inconsistently picked up by patients, particularly patients at high risk of overdose seen in the ED.[52,53] Providers and hospitals have attempted to overcome this obstacle by dispensing naloxone directly to patients while in the ED.[54] Implementation barriers exist, including training, costs, means of distribution, and patient education, but the idea may be a novel and successful approach in reducing overdose deaths.[54–56] There are reimbursement barriers related to naloxone *dispensed but not administered* in the ED, further impeding distribution and underscoring the need for system-level change to advance public health initiatives.[55,56] In addition, state laws may limit dispensing of medications from inpatient pharmacies.

CLINICS CARE POINTS

- Naloxone is an effective medication for opioid overdose reversal.
- Naloxone can be dispensed without a prescription in all states via standing order.
- The cost of naloxone continues to be a barrier to its community distribution.
- Co-prescribing naloxone with opioids and dispensing take-home naloxone from EDs aim to increase naloxone access, though there are barriers to both practices.
- The people most likely to save a life with naloxone are people who use opioids themselves—as such, they are a priority population to receive naloxone.

Looking Forward

This article's aim is to provide primary care providers with pertinent updates on opioid use and chronic pain management. The number of overdose deaths caused by opioids continues to increase, with ultra-potent fentanyl analogs saturating the drug supply. Although fentanyl is currently used primarily via inhalation, it is not unreasonable to expect a transition to intravenous fentanyl use in the coming years. This represents an enormous increase in risk to an already hazardous practice.

In the face of this challenging landscape, the medical community must continue to implement the essential practice of harm reduction. Harm reduction aims to mitigate the negative consequences of risks of drug use without condemning or endorsing said use. Examples of harm reduction include syringe access programs, overdose prevention centers, and fentanyl testing strips.[57] Harm reduction practices have a proven track record of reducing infectious disease transmission, decreased risk of overdose, and enhanced engagement in treatment.

The medical community must address opioid initiation and use across the spectrum of prevention.[58] The prevention of opioid use initiation and promotion of harm reduction practices—especially to high-risk populations—using a multilevel approach may decrease negative outcomes at a public health level while decreasing stigma around drug use as well. The coordinated implementation of primary, secondary, and tertiary prevention strategies will mitigate the impact of adverse outcomes associated with opioid use. The American College of Preventive Medicine strongly supports this approach and endorses population-level interventions.[58]

As health care providers, we must strive to keep our patients safe and healthy using every available tool in our toolkit. We hope that this review helps the reader accomplish this goal.

DISCLOSURE

The authors report no actual or perceived conflicts of interest. The viewpoints presented in this article represent the opinion of the authors and do not reflect the position of their employers. This article has not been published elsewhere.

AUTHOR CONTRIBUTIONS

E. Salisbury-Afshar, D.T. Coyle, and T. Locke conceptualized the initial commentary. T. Locke conducted supporting research and authored the article. E. Salisbury-Afshar, D.T. Coyle, and T. Locke provided critical feedback and contributed to the writing of the article.

ACKNOWLEDGMENTS

This work was supported by the University of Colorado School of Medicine, United States and the University of Wisconsin School of Medicine and Public Health, United States.

REFERENCES

1. Dennen AC, Blum K, Braverman RE, et al. How to Combat the Global Opioid Crisis. CPQ Neurol Psychol 2023;5(4):93.
2. Spencer MR, Miniño AM, Warner M. Drug overdose deaths in the United States, 2001–2021. NCHS Data Brief, no 457. Hyattsville, MD: National Center for Health Statistics; 2022. https://doi.org/10.15620/cdc:122556.

3. Dowell D, Haegerich TM, Chou R. CDC Guideline for Prescribing Opioids for Chronic Pain — United States, 2016. MMWR Recomm Rep (Morb Mortal Wkly Rep) 2016;65(No. RR-1):1–49.

4. Coyle DT, Pratt CY, Ocran-Appiah J, et al. Opioid analgesic dose and the risk of misuse, overdose, and death: A narrative review. Pharmacoepidemiol Drug Saf 2018 May;27(5):464–72.

5. Dowell D, Ragan KR, Jones CM, et al. CDC Clinical Practice Guideline for Prescribing Opioids for Pain — United States, 2022. MMWR Recomm Rep (Morb Mortal Wkly Rep) 2022;71(No. RR-3):1–95.

6. Methadone Take-Home Flexibilities Extension Guidance. U.S. Department of Health and Human Services, Substance Abuse and Mental Health Services Administration. https://www.samhsa.gov/medications-substance-use-disorders/statutes-regulations-guidelines/methadone-guidance#:~:text=On%20March%2016%2C%202020%2C%20SAMHSA,14%20days%20of%20Take%2DHome. Accessed 25 Jan 2023.

7. Amram O, Amiri S, Panwala V, et al. The impact of relaxation of methadone take-home protocols on treatment outcomes in the COVID-19 era. Am J Drug Alcohol Abuse 2021;47(6):722–9.

8. Krawczyk N, Rivera B, Levin E, et al. Synthesising evidence of the effects of COVID-19 regulatory changes on methadone treatment for opioid use disorder: implications for policy. Lancet Public Health 2023;8:e238–46.

9. SAMHSA Extends the Methadone Take-Home Flexibility for One Year While Working Toward a Permanent Solution. U.S. Department of Health and Human Services, Substance Abuse and Mental Health Services Administration from https://www.samhsa.gov/newsroom/press-announcements/202111181000. Accessed 26 Jan 2023.

10. Joudrey PJ, Bart G, Brooner RK, et al. Research priorities for expanding access to methadone treatment for opioid use disorder in the United States: A National Institute on Drug Abuse Center for Clinical Trials Network Task Force report. Subst Abus 2021;42(3):245–54 [Erratum in: Subst Abus. 2022;43(1):691].

11. Chan B, Bougatsos C, Priest KC, et al. Opioid treatment programs, telemedicine and COVID-19: A scoping review. Subst Abus 2022;43(1):539–46.

12. Jones CM, Shoff C, Hodges K, et al. Receipt of Telehealth Services, Receipt and Retention of Medications for Opioid Use Disorder, and Medically Treated Overdose Among Medicare Beneficiaries Before and During the COVID-19 Pandemic. JAMA Psychiatr 2022;79(10):981–92.

13. Hallgren KA, Darnton J, Soth S, et al. Acceptability, feasibility, and outcomes of a clinical pilot program for video observation of methadone take-home dosing during the COVID-19 pandemic. J Subst Abuse Treat 2022;143:108896.

14. Beardsley K, Wish ED, Fitzelle DB, et al. Distance traveled to outpatient drug treatment and client retention. J Subst Abuse Treat 2003;25(4):279–85.

15. Registration Requirements for Narcotic Treatment Programs With Mobile Components. Drug Enforcement Administration, Department of Justice. (Federal Register, The Daily Journal of the United States Government) Document Citation 2021; 86 FR 33861.

16. Consolidated Appropriations Act of 2023. Available at https://www.appropriations.senate.gov/imo/media/doc/JRQ121922.PDF. Accessed on 1 Mar 2023.

17. Drug Enforcement Administration, Department of Justice; 12 Jan 2023. https://www.deadiversion.usdoj.gov/pubs/docs/A-23-0020-Dear-Registrant-Letter-Signed.pdf. Accessed 13 Mar 2023.

18. Herring AA, Vosooghi AA, Luftig J, et al. High-Dose Buprenorphine Induction in the Emergency Department for Treatment of Opioid Use Disorder. JAMA Netw Open 2021;4(7):e2117128.

19. Spadaro A, Faude S, Perrone J, et al. Precipitated opioid withdrawal after buprenorphine administration in patients presenting to the emergency department: A case series. J Am Coll Emerg Physicians Open 2023;4(1):e12880.

20. Ahmed S, Bhivandkar S, Lonergan BB, et al. Microinduction of Buprenorphine/Naloxone: A Review of the Literature. Am J Addict 2021;30:305–15.

21. Ciccarone D. The rise of illicit fentanyls, stimulants and the fourth wave of the opioid overdose crisis. Curr Opin Psychiatry 2021;34(4):344–50.

22. McNeil R, Puri N, Boyd J, et al. Understanding concurrent stimulant use among people on methadone: A qualitative study. Drug Alcohol Rev 2020;39(3):209–15.

23. Ellis MS, Kasper ZA, Cicero TJ. Twin epidemics: The surging rise of methamphetamine use in chronic opioid users. Drug Alcohol Depend 2018;193:14–20.

24. Substance Abuse and Mental Health Services Administration (SAMHSA). Treatment of stimulant use disorders. SAMHSA publication No. PEP20-06-01-001. Rockville, MD: National Mental Health and Substance Use Policy Laboratory; 2020. Substance Abuse and Mental Health Services Administration.

25. Brown HD, DeFulio A. Contingency management for the treatment of methamphetamine use disorder: A systematic review. Drug Alcohol Depend 2020;216:108307.

26. Petry NM. Contingency management treatments: controversies and challenges. Addiction 2010;105(9):1507–9.

27. Bentzley BS, Han SS, Neuner S, et al. Comparison of Treatments for Cocaine Use Disorder Among Adults: A Systematic Review and Meta-analysis. JAMA Netw Open 2021;4(5):e218049.

28. AshaRani PV, Hombali A, Seow E, et al. Non-pharmacological interventions for methamphetamine use disorder: a systematic review. Drug Alcohol Depend 2020;212:108060.

29. Murphy SM, McDonell MG, McPherson S, et al. An economic evaluation of a contingency-management intervention for stimulant use among community mental health patients with serious mental illness. Drug Alcohol Depend 2015;153:293–9.

30. Kaiser Family Foundation. Medicaid Waiver Tracker: Approved and Pending Section 1115 Waivers by State. Available at: https://www.kff.org/medicaid/issue-brief/medicaid-waiver-tracker-approved-and-pending-section-1115-waivers-by-state/. Accessed 13 Mar 2023.

31. Montana Expanding Stimulant Use Disorder Treatment. Montana Department of Public Health and Human Services Available at: https://dphhs.mt.gov/News/2021/09/StimulantUseDisorder. Accessed 3 Feb 2023.

32. Recovery Incentives Program: California's Contingency Management Benefit. Department of Healthcare Services. Available at: https://www.dhcs.ca.gov/Pages/DMC-ODS-Contingency-Management.aspx. Accessed 2 Feb 2023.

33. California Health Care Foundation Issue Brief. Treating Stimulant Use Disorder: CalAIM's Contingency Management Pilot. Available at: https://www.chcf.org/wp-content/uploads/2022/05/TreatingStimulantUseDisorderCalAIMsContingencyMgmtPilot.pdf. Access 13 Mar 2023.

34. Contingency Management (CM) project. Washington State Health Authority Available at: https://www.hca.wa.gov/assets/program/contingency-mangement-fact-sheet.pdf. Accessed 3 Feb, 2023

35. West Virginia Medicaid Section 1115 Waiver Demonstration: Evolving West Virginia Medicaid's Behavioral Health Continuum of Care Available at: 12.1.21.pdf">https://dhhr.wv.gov/bms/Public%20Notices/Documents/20211201_SUD_Waiver_Extension_Application_Final%20Version%2012.1.21.pdf. Accessed 28 Feb 2023.
36. Gangal NS, Hincapie AL, Jandarov R, et al. Association between a state law allowing pharmacists to dispense naloxone without a prescription and naloxone dispensing rates. JAMA Netw Open 2020;3(1):e1920310.
37. Gertner AK, Domino ME, Davis CS. Do naloxone access laws increase outpatient naloxone prescriptions? Evidence from Medicaid. Drug Alcohol Depend 2018; 190:37–41.
38. Pharmacists' Role in Naloxone Dispensing. Centers for Disease Control and Prevention National Center for Injury Prevention and Control. Available at: https://www.cdc.gov/opioids/naloxone/factsheets/pdf/Naloxone_FactSheet_Pharmacists.pdf. Accessed 13 Mar 2023.
39. Silverman E. A drug maker boosted the price of its opioid-overdose antidote by 600 percent, and taxpayers suffered. Stat News 2018;19. Available at: https://www.statnews.com/pharmalot/2018/11/19/kaleo-opioid-antidote-price-probe/. Accessed 13 March, 2023.
40. US Department of Justice. Kaleo Inc. Agrees to Pay $12.7 Million to Resolve Allegations of False Claims for Anti-Overdose Drug. Available at: https://www.justice.gov/opa/pr/kal-o-inc-agrees-pay-127-million-resolve-allegations-false-claims-anti-overdose-drug. Accessed 13 March 2023.
41. Peet ED, Powell D, Pacula RL. Trends in out-of-pocket costs for naloxone by drug brand and payer in the US, 2010-2018. JAMA Health Forum 2022;3(8):e222663.
42. Spivey CA, Wilder A, Chisholm-Burns MA, et al. Evaluation of naloxone access, pricing, and barriers to dispensing in Tennessee retail community pharmacies. J Am Pharm Assoc 2003 2020;60(5):694–701.
43. Clemans-Cope L. Naloxone Products and Their Pricing in Medicaid, 2010-2018. Urban Institute. Available at: https://www.urban.org/sites/default/files/publication/102769/naloxone-products-and-their-pricing-in-medicaid-2010-18.pdf,   Accessed 7 February 2023.
44. Roberts AW, Look KA, Trull G, et al. Medicaid prescription limits and their implications for naloxone accessibility. Drug Alcohol Depend 2021;218:108355.
45. Facher L. FDA advisers recommend approval of over-the-counter naloxone to fight opioid overdose. Stat News 2023;15. Available at: https://www.statnews.com/2023/02/15/naloxone-otc-opioisa-fda-panel-recommends/#:~:text=FDA%20advisers%20recommend%20approval%20of,naloxone%20to%20fight%20opioid%20overdose&text=A%20government%20advisory%20committee%20voted,and%20distributed%20without%20a%20prescription. Accessed 28 February, 2023.
46. Naloxone Access: Summary of State Laws. Legislative Analysis and Public Policy Association   Available   at: Access-Summary-of-State-Laws.pdf">http://legislativeanalysis.org/wp-content/uploads/2023/02/Naloxone-Access-Summary-of-State-Laws.pdf, Accessed 7 February, 2023.
47. NEXT Distro Stay Alive, Stay Safe. Next Distro. Available at: https://nextdistro.org/naloxone. Accessed 7 February 2023.
48. Torres-Leguizamon M, Favaro J, Coello D, Reynaud EG, Nefau T, Duplessy C. Remote harm reduction services are key solutions to reduce the impact of COVID-19-like crises on people who use drugs: evidence from two independent structures in France and in the USA. Harm Reduct J 2023;20(1):1.

49. Jones CM, Compton W, Vythilingam M, et al. Naloxone Co-prescribing to Patients Receiving Prescription Opioids in the Medicare Part D Program, United States, 2016-2017. JAMA 2019;322(5):462–4.
50. Stein BD, Smart R, Jones CM, et al. Individual and Community Factors Associated with Naloxone Co-prescribing Among Long-term Opioid Patients: A Retrospective Analysis. J Gen Intern Med 2021;36(10):2952–7.
51. Duska M, Rhoads JM, Saunders EC, et al. State naloxone co-prescribing laws show mixed effects on overdose mortality rates. Drug Science, Policy and Law 2022;8.
52. Weiner SG, Hoppe JA. Prescribing Naloxone to High-Risk Patients in the Emergency Department: Is it Enough? Jt Comm J Qual Patient Saf 2021;47(6):340–2.
53. Verdier M, Routsolias J, Aks S. Naloxone Prescriptions from the Emergency Department: An Initiative in Evolution. Am J Emer Med 2019;37:164–5.
54. Gunn AH, Smothers ZPW, Schramm-Sapyta N, et al. The emergency department as an opportunity for naloxone distribution. West J Emerg Med 2018;19(6):1036–42.
55. Moore PQ, Cheema N, Celmins LE, et al. Point-of-care naloxone distribution in the emergency department: a pilot study. Am J Health Syst Pharm 2021;78(4):360–6.
56. Eswaran V, Allen KC, Bottari DC, et al. Take-home naloxone program implementation: lessons learned from seven Chicago-area hospitals. Ann Emerg Med 2020;76(3):318–27.
57. Centers for Disease Control and Prevention. Harm Reduction Available at: https://www.cdc.gov/drugoverdose/od2a/case-studies/harm-reduction.html. Accessed 13 Mar 2023.
58. Livingston CJ, Berenji M, Titus TM, et al. American College of Preventive Medicine: Addressing the Opioid Epidemic Through a Prevention Framework. Am J Prev Med 2022;63(3):454–65.

Brief Action Planning in Health and Health Care

A Scoping Review

Yuri Jadotte, MD, PhD, MPH[a,b,*], Benjamin Buchholz, MPH[c],
William Carroll, MD[d], Deirdra Frum-Vassallo, PhD[e],
Janelle MacPherson[f], Steven Cole, MD, MA[f,g,h,i]

KEYWORDS

- Brief action planning • Motivational interviewing • Self-management support
- Health behavior change • Mental health • Prevention

KEY POINTS

- Brief action planning (BAP) facilitates patient self-management, health behavior change, and health coaching, to optimize health promotion and disease prevention.
- Using a comprehensive search strategy, this scoping review identified 143 relevant papers and clarifies the extent and type of evidence available about BAP to date.
- BAP has been applied primarily in North America, within community settings, and evaluated using relatively high-level research designs.
- BAP has mostly been used for health care, and is mostly grounded within the framework of motivational interviewing, as originally intended.
- The fidelity of BAP remains unclear or underreported, regardless of which fidelity domain is examined.

[a] Department of Family, Population, and Preventive Medicine, Renaissance School of Medicine, Stony Brook University, Stony Brook, NY, USA; [b] Northeast Institute for Evidence Synthesis and Translation, Division of Nursing Science, School of Nursing, Rutgers University, Newark NJ, USA; [c] Sickle Cell Center of Excellence, College of Medicine, Howard University, Washington, DC, USA; [d] Department of Medicine, David Geffen School of Medicine, University of California, Los Angeles CA, USA; [e] Health Promotion Disease Prevention, Northport VA Medical Center, Northport, NY, USA; [f] BAP Professional Network, US; [g] Department of Psychiatry, Renaissance School of Medicine, Stony Brook University, Stony Brook, NY, USA; [h] Department of Scientific Education, Zucker SOM at Hofstra/Northwell, Hempstead, NY, USA; [i] Department of Psychiatry, Zucker SOM at Hofstra/Northwell, Hempstead, NY, USA
* Corresponding author. Health Sciences Center, Stony Brook University, Level 3, Room 087, Stony Brook, NY 11794
E-mail address: yuri.jadotte@stonybrookmedicine.edu

Med Clin N Am 107 (2023) 1047–1096
https://doi.org/10.1016/j.mcna.2023.06.018

INTRODUCTION

There is widespread agreement in the literature that the top 2 conditions that cause death both globally and regionally are ischemic heart disease and cerebrovascular disease.[1] However, it is also known that tobacco use, poor nutrition, inadequate physical activity, and the consumption of alcohol are the leading actual causes of death,[2] and that these factors are preventable, modifiable, and amenable to health behavior change interventions.[3] Brief action planning (BAP) is a novel, teachable, feasible, and potentially high-fidelity approach to support patient self-management, facilitate health behavior change, and enhance health coaching. Originally conceptualized circa 2002 by one of the authors of this review (SC), as "ultra-brief personal action planning," and subsequently with contributions from others renamed BAP,[4] it was designed to facilitate the self-management support component of the chronic care model for health care transformation.[5] An important goal is to facilitate the uptake by primary care and mental health providers of a medical interviewing approach that transcends collecting information and engages the patient in action toward self-management and sustainable health behavior change for health promotion and disease prevention.[4]

The approach is considered teachable for several reasons. First, it consists of 8 competencies that aim to help clinicians acquire a set of techniques that can then be applied immediately to subsequent patient care or client cases. Second, the basic structure can be presented in a single didactic session, with asynchronous self-directed online modules available to facilitate this teaching. However, skilled use of BAP also requires the presence of good rapport (eg, engagement, connection) as well as elements of the Spirit of Motivational Interviewing (eg, autonomy support, partnership, and empowerment). These are considerably more difficult to master than the straightforward competencies themselves, so teaching and learning BAP is often best conceptualized as occurring in stages. Recitation of the words tied to the core competencies can be learned and even utilized after a single session exposure. However, the effectiveness with which these competencies can be applied clinically, and whether they are being utilized with the suggested values and attitudes of the "Spirit of MI," has not yet been clarified. Third, there is evidence that BAP can be integrated into existing teaching models for physicians and other health professionals aiming to teach their trainees methods for encouraging patient and client health behavior change.[6–8] Lastly, it does not require an extensive curriculum or training, unlike the closely related approach of Motivational Interviewing (MI), an older and more common methodology in the fields of health behavior change, self-management, and health coaching.

BAP is grounded in the principles and practice of MI. Both approaches place a high value on patient engagement and aim to train clinicians to use active listening, open-ended and reflective communication, as well as develop an orientation toward promoting change talk (ie, verbal communication from the patient or client that favors making a change) and minimizing sustain talk (ie, verbal communication from the patient or client that favors the status quo of not making a change). Moreover, BAP is explicitly informed by the "Spirit of MI," emphasizing the principles of partnership, acceptance/autonomy, compassion, and evocation.[4] MI as an approach to help patients and clients change their health behaviors has been studied extensively and has been found to be effective via a wide body of literature.[9,10] Tools, approaches, and methods for the application of BAP in clinical practice are widely available from a variety of sources, including peer-reviewed published articles[4,6] and organizational websites.[11,12]

The effectiveness of complex behavioral interventions, such as MI, has been found to vary widely across studies, sites, and providers, and has been linked to the fidelity of the treatment intervention.[13] Fidelity is defined as the degree of exactness with which something is copied or reproduced.[14] In the realm of health and health care, this is generally understood to mean the degree to which an intervention is delivered at the individual patient care level, or implemented at a systems level, relative to an established intervention that is known to be effective.[15] The notion of effectiveness is grounded in the assumptions of evidence-based decision-making, which are that high-quality primary research studies (ie, randomized controlled trials) have shown that an intervention has a statistically measurable and clinically significant effect, and that the effect of the intervention has been verified further via a synthesis of the primary research studies (ie, systematic review [SR] with meta-analysis [MA]). A search of the Cochrane Library, JBI Evidence Synthesis, and Google Scholar has not identified an SR of the effects of BAP. However, a search of the PROSPERO data-base has identified a protocol on this topic,[16] suggesting the work of assessing the effectiveness of BAP to date is actively being undertaken.

While the literature suggests that BAP has been widely adopted in different fields,[4,17–19] the ways in which BAP is being applied in practice is unclear. For example, it is unknown whether each of the 8 competencies of BAP are being taught or applied as originally devised. Clinicians launch BAP with Question One: "Is there anything you'd like to do for your health in the next week or two?" This question is designed to be a grammatically closed-ended but generative and conceptually open question[20] that typically produces "change talk" (ie, speech that favors the direction of behavior change). Context-relevant adaptations of Question One are also considered fully aligned and acceptable BAP practice. For example, in the context of an ongoing discussion about smoking, a clinician could launch BAP, with a context-relevant version of Question One, for example, "I'm wondering now that we've been discussing your feelings about smoking and stopping smoking, whether you feel like you'd like to go ahead and make a plan about stopping smoking?"

Yet the authors find, based on their own pedagogic practice in BAP, that clinicians, trainees, and students newly exposed to BAP often modify this question as they attempt to emulate the approach or adapt it to fit other medical interviewing approaches (eg, "what would you like to work on today?"). In addition, although BAP was originally grounded in the "Spirit of MI," its algorithmic approach may lend itself to the adaptation or adoption of BAP to fit within other health counseling traditions, theoretic paradigms or approaches other than MI. Also, not much is known about how BAP effectiveness varies by small modifications in how the core competencies are delivered in practice.

Finally, the extent to which BAP has been adopted in the scholarly practice of different disciplines or professions is not known. A Google search for the exact term "brief action planning" on January 31, 2023, yielded 9280 results, suggesting that there is widespread adoption of at least this terminology in the searchable online ether. But the degree to which this terminological presence of BAP translates into scholarly work on BAP that is validated, replicable, and useable in pedagogic or clinical practice contexts is undetermined. Specifically, within the contexts of health and health care, the conceptual/theoretic grounding of BAP, and the applications of BAP in real world settings, in addition to the fidelity of its delivery or implementation, are currently unknown. Addressing these aspects is critical to facilitating the use of BAP as a health behavior change approach that optimizes health promotion and disease prevention.

A search of the Cochrane Library, JBI Evidence Synthesis, and Google Scholar has not identified a scoping review (ScR) or protocol on this topic. The objective of this scoping review is to explore the extent and type of evidence that exist in the literature regarding the use of BAP within the context of health and health care.

REVIEW QUESTION

The review question is: what is the extent and type of evidence that exists in the literature regarding the use of BAP within the context of health and health care?

INCLUSION CRITERIA
Participants

Participants in this review were either adults or children, regardless of their professional status (eg, students or non-students, faculty, staff, clinical personnel, patients, educators, administrators), age, gender, race/ethnicity, sexual orientation, profession, specialty, and mental or physical health conditions.

Concept

The review considered articles that included BAP in any format (eg, as an algorithm for guiding planning within the context of or in the absence of MI, as a component of MI, as a research intervention, an educational program, or a practice/systems-based tool or technique for quality improvement).

Context

The context of interest is health or health care. However, articles that did not fit this context from the clinical practice standpoint were not excluded from the review. While the emphasis is on health and health care, it is critical to examine the full breadth of contexts within health and health care where BAP has been used to date in order to answer the review question. For example, health care research, health care education, public health research, and public health education were all considered valid contexts, given their relevance to the broader context of health and health care writ large.

Types of Sources

This scoping review considered both experimental and quasi-experimental study designs including randomized controlled trials, non-randomized controlled trials, before and after studies and interrupted time-series studies. In addition, analytical observational studies including prospective and retrospective cohort studies, case-control studies and analytical cross-sectional studies were considered for inclusion. This review also considered descriptive observational study designs including case series, individual case reports, and descriptive cross-sectional studies for inclusion.

Qualitative studies were also considered that focus on textual data including, but not limited to, designs such as phenomenology, grounded theory, ethnography, qualitative description, action research, and feminist research. In addition, systematic reviews and other forms of evidence synthesis (eg, narrative/traditional literature reviews) that met the inclusion criteria were also considered, depending on the research question. Text and opinion papers were also considered for inclusion in this scoping review. Articles were not excluded based on methodology.

METHODS

The proposed scoping review was conducted in accordance with the JBI methodology for scoping reviews.[21,22] This scoping review protocol was registered a priori in the Open Science Framework (OSF) project registry.[23]

Search Strategy

This review utilized a three-step search strategy to identify both published and unpublished studies. First an initial limited search of MEDLINE (PubMed) and CINAHL (EBSCO) was undertaken to identify articles on the topic. The text words contained in the titles and abstracts of relevant articles, and the index terms used to describe the articles were used to develop a full search strategy for 12 databases listed in Appendix 1. Due to the high specificity of the concept under study, the search strategy consisted of the use of a single term that needed to appear verbatim in each article for it to be eligible for inclusion (ie, brief action planning). Articles that did not use this term were not considered in this search, since they did not adhere to this basic and fundamental aspect of BAP.

In addition, keywords related to the population or context were considered too nonspecific and unlikely to yield meaningful results. For example, the key words "adult" and "children" would result in millions of irrelevant articles, while the key words "health" and "health care" would not only result in millions of irrelevant articles, but they would also potentially exclude valuable scholarship on BAP that was done in other related contexts, such as education, thereby precluding the synthesis of an evidence map situating BAP in the general literature. The search strategy, including all identified keywords and index terms, was adapted for each included database and/or information source. The reference list of all included sources of evidence was screened for additional studies. Studies published in any language were included and recorded at the title and abstract phase, as long as the records of these were in English, but only English language articles were included at the full-text level. There were no date limitations. No authors of articles were contacted to retrieve data that was not available in the online databases due to time and resource constraints.

Google Scholar was searched to identify unpublished studies. Additional sources of unpublished studies and gray literature included Clinicaltrials.gov, the WHO international clinical trials registry platform, and the following organizations' websites: the American Psychiatric Association (APA) including the Mental Health Services Conference (IPS); the American Psychological Association; the Academy of Consultation-Liaison Psychiatry (ACLP); the American College of Physicians (ACP); the New York Chapter of the American College of Physicians (NYACP); the Motivational Interviewing Network of Trainers (MINT) including the International Conference on Motivational Interviewing (ICMI); the Institute for Healthcare Improvement (IHI); the Centers for Disease Control and Prevention (CDC); the Health Resources and Services Administration (HRSA); the Substance Abuse and Mental Health Services Administration (SAMHSA); and the Indian Health Service (IHS). The NYACP site was searched because BAP was founded by one of the authors (SC) during his appointments at academic institutions in NY.

Study/Source of Evidence Selection

Following the search, all identified citations were collated and uploaded into EndNote version 20/y 2023 (Clarivate Analytics, PA, USA) with all readily identifiable duplicate records removed. Following a pilot test, titles and abstracts were then screened by two or more independent reviewers for assessment against the inclusion criteria for the review. Potentially relevant sources were retrieved in full. The full text of each selected citation was assessed in detail against the inclusion criteria by two or more independent reviewers. Reasons for exclusion of studies or other sources of evidence at full-text review that did not meet the inclusion criteria were recorded and reported. Any disagreements that arose between the reviewers at each stage of the selection process were resolved through discussion, or with an additional reviewer. The results of the search and the study inclusion process are reported in full in this final scoping review report and presented in a Preferred Reporting Items for Systematic Reviews and Meta-analyses extension for scoping review (PRISMA-ScR) flow diagram.[24,25]

Data Extraction

Data were extracted from papers included in the scoping review by two independent reviewers using the JBI data extraction tool for ScR,[21,22] modified by the reviewers to better suit the needs of this review. The modified tool excludes the "scoping review details" and the "inclusion/exclusion criteria" items in the original JBI data extraction tool as these are already stated in the protocol and will not result in the capture of useful data from the included studies. In addition, the results section of the tool was modified to specify the 4 domains of information sought from the included studies. The data extracted included specific details about the participants, concept, context, study methods, and key findings relevant to the review question. In extracting data on the fidelity of BAP from the included papers, we adhered to the recommendations from a prior scoping review that defined the 4 key elements of fidelity in intervention research studies: design, training, monitoring intervention delivery, and monitoring intervention receipt.[15] We also included an additional domain of "Other aspects of fidelity" to capture any element of fidelity that could not be easily classified in one of the other 4 domains.

The data extraction form is provided in Appendix 2. No modifications to the data extraction form were necessary during the process of extracting data from each included evidence source. Any disagreements that arose between the reviewers were resolved through discussion, or with an additional reviewer. No authors of papers were contacted to request missing or additional data due to time and resource constraints, and sensitivity analyses showed that missing data had no meaningful influence on the interpretation of the results.

Data Analysis and Presentation

The data extracted from the included studies are presented in graphs, charts, tables, and diagrams, with the goal of developing evidence gap maps[26] that help to answer the research question, by demonstrating the extent to which BAP has been applied in different contexts, professions or disciplines, and by identifying the elements of fidelity to BAP (eg, whether all 8 competencies were taught, whether any elements of the BAP algorithm were modified, and whether MI was integrated into BAP or vice versa and how this was accomplished), and the conceptual/theoretic foundations that BAP was grounded in within the included articles. A narrative summary accompanies the graphed, charted, tabulated, and diagrammed results to describe how the results relate to the reviews objective and question.

RESULTS
Study Inclusion

The search strategy identified 508 papers from the databases and registers and 42 papers from other literature sources, as shown in **Fig. 1**. De-duplication using EndNote removed 170 records, resulting in 380 records that were eligible for screening. Of those, 76 were excluded by title and abstract, followed by an additional 65 that were further excluded as a full-text paper could not be retrieved after substantive attempts by the authorship team. Of the 239 full-text articles retrieved, 96 were excluded on the following bases: 78 did not address the concept of BAP, 14 were duplicate

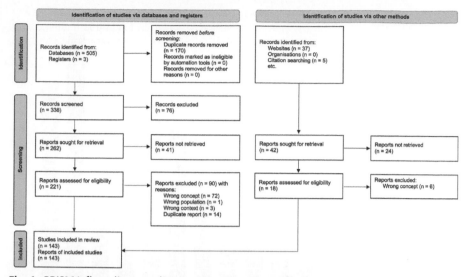

Fig. 1. PRISMA flow diagram. (Source: Page MJ, McKenzie JE, Bossuyt PM et al. The PRISMA 2020 statement: an updated guideline for reporting systematic reviews. BMJ 2021;372: n71. Doi: 10.1136/bmj. n71.)

reports of the studies already included, 3 did not address any identifiable context of relevance (eg, health, health care, or education), and 1 was not about either adults or children. Appendix 3 lists the citations for the 96 articles excluded by full-text review with a reason for exclusion provided for each article. The remaining 143 articles were included in this review.

Characteristics of Included Studies

The articles were published between the years 2006 and 2023, with the great majority being published between 2012 and 2022. **Fig. 2** illustrates a distribution of articles related to BAP ranked by year of publication. Most articles using BAP originate from North America (ie, 46% in the USA, and 42% in Canada), with the remaining articles coming from a small number of other countries or regions (ie, 5% in the UK, 4% from multiple countries, and 1% each from Australia, Iran, Mexico, and Germany). **Fig. 3** illustrates these geographic proportions.

Nearly a third (29%) of all participants experiencing BAP were located in community settings, meaning that they were members of the general public, as compared to patients in a clinic setting, which represented a quarter of sites of BAP application (25%). School settings are also well represented in the literature on BAP, ranking 3rd among the identifiable sites at 13% of articles, while the setting was not specified in 15% of articles. The remaining sites are represented in single digits: 9% in various combinations of clinic, hospital, and community settings; 6% in health systems writ large; 2% in hospitals; and only 1% in research settings. **Fig. 4** depicts the sites/settings where participants in BAP were located.

Lastly, there is wide variation in the types of evidence sources or study designs that the articles used with regards to BAP. Nearly a fifth (19%) of the articles were traditional parallel group randomized controlled trials or protocols for such trials, with an additional 6% being quasi-experimental (pre-test/post-test designs), 3% cluster randomized controlled trials, and 1% having an unspecified clinical trial design. Observational study designs were the 2nd most well-represented group, including 4%

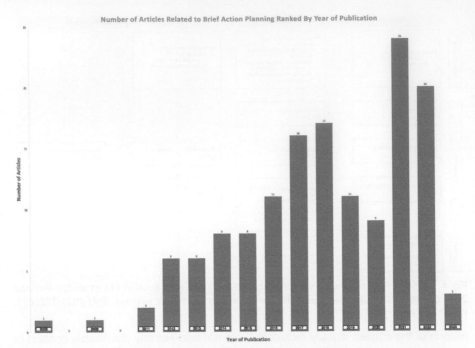

Fig. 2. Distribution of articles related to BAP by year of publication.

prospective cohorts, 6% retrospective cohorts, and 2% cross-sectional descriptive designs. Literature reviews were the 3rd most common type of article: 6% traditional literature reviews, 2% systematic reviews, and 2% scoping reviews. Different types of preliminary or early studies have also been conducted, including pilot studies (5%), and feasibility studies (3%). A large diversity of additional types of evidence sources were also used but in smaller proportions, as illustrated in **Fig. 5**. A table detailing the characteristics of all included studies and a list of citations for these studies are provided in Appendix 4.

Review Findings

The review findings center around 4 aspects of BAP: the context of the application of BAP, the conceptual grounding of BAP, the discipline or profession applying BAP, and the fidelity of BAP. As demonstrated in **Fig. 6**, covering 77% of all articles, BAP has been applied primarily in health care contexts, which is where the clinical (ie, acute or chronic disease) care of patients takes place. General health contexts represent 13% of articles. These include public health and community health contexts. Educational settings constitute the remainder of settings, with medical education being the most identifiable subtype of education in this group.

As shown in **Fig. 7**, only 44% of articles specified the conceptual or theoretic framework that grounded their application of BAP. Of those, MI was by far the most well represented, at 63% of articles reporting a theoretic framework. Some articles reported BAP as its own theoretic framework, while others reported multiple theories (8% each). These theories included: action planning (5%), self-management support (5%), peer support (3%), shared decision-making (3%), brief counseling (1.5%), theory of planned behavior (1.5%), and the transtheoretical model (1.5%).

Proportion of Articles Related to BAP by Country/Region of Application

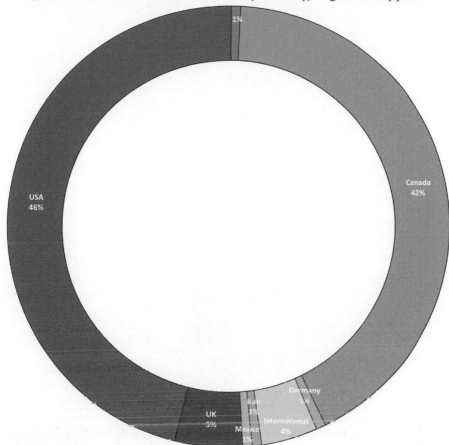

☐ Australia ☐ Canada ☐ Germany ☐ International ☐ Iran ☐ Mexico ■ UK ■ USA

Fig. 3. Country or region of application of BAP.

Context/Site of BAP Application

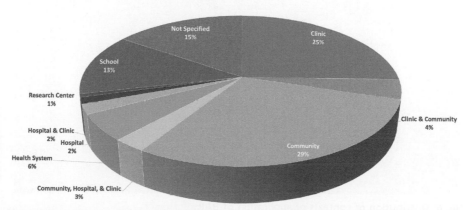

Fig. 4. Sites/settings where participants in BAP were located.

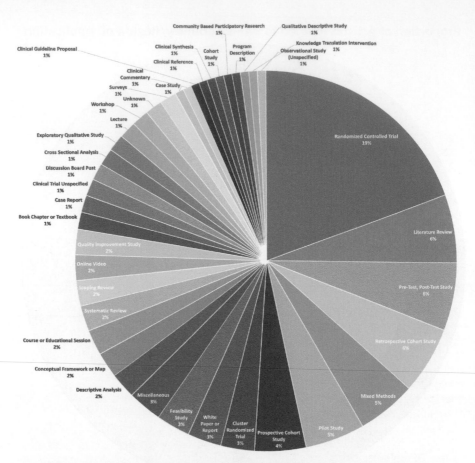

Types of Evidence Source/Study Design of BAP Application

Fig. 5. Types of evidence sources/study designs.

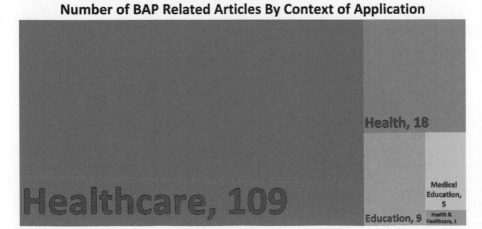

Number of BAP Related Articles By Context of Application

Fig. 6. Distribution of contexts of application of BAP.

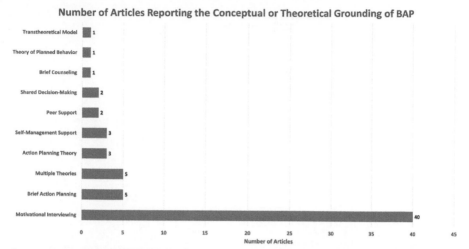

Fig. 7. Conceptual grounding of BAP.

The disciplines or professions that have applied BAP have also been diverse. While multiple disciplines collaborating represented the largest group of studies (23%), physical therapy is the most well represented profession to date in the literature, followed by primary care (14%), though the specific primary care professions could not be disaggregated. Other well represented professions include health coaching (8%), preventive medicine (5%), community health education (5%), and chiropractic (5%). Other professions are also represented, but at smaller proportions (1%–2%), as shown in **Fig. 8**.

At least one aspect of fidelity of BAP was mentioned in up to 52% of articles, and only 2 of the 5 identified domains of fidelity were captured on average in each of these articles. Of the articles that did measure some aspect of fidelity, the following are the proportions represented: 62% for BAP design, 55% for BAP training, 36% for BAP delivery, 41% for BAP receipt, and 4% for miscellaneous aspects of fidelity.

DISCUSSION

This scoping review provides a map of the literature on when, where, how, and why BAP has been applied to date. One critical finding is that while BAP has been presented using a variety of types of study designs or scholarly evaluations, a large proportion of these have been high-level evidence for effectiveness, including both experimental and observational research. As recommended in guidelines for scoping reviews, this scoping review did not assess the methodological quality of the included studies,[22] as this was not relevant to the objectives of this scoping review or most scoping reviews. This suggests that the literature may now be ripe for the conduct of a systematic review of this body of evidence on the application of BAP.

Of note, a limitation is that this scoping review did not pursue non-academic and non-organizational sources of evidence (eg, evidence from non-profit groups such as the Center for Collaboration, Motivation and Innovation, blog posts not affiliated with a known organization that works in this field such as the Motivational Interviewing Network of Trainers, and so forth). This may be an area to explore in future research studies to map the literature more comprehensively on the application of BAP. However, the choice to exclude these evidence sources is a delimitation of this review,

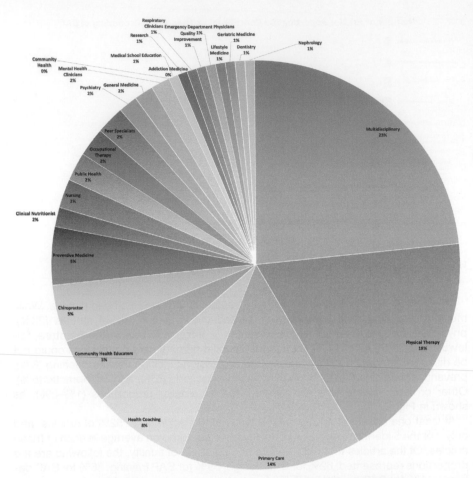

Discipline or Profession of BAP Application

Fig. 8. Disciplines or professions that have used BAP as recorded in the literature.

based on the pre-specified aim to map the terminological presence of BAP in scholarly works that are validated, replicable, and useable in pedagogic or clinical practice contexts. In addition, while the review aimed to identify the professions and disciplines that have utilized BAP to date, it became apparent that it would have been beneficial to extract data on the clinical topics where BAP has been used. Unfortunately, this would have been a substantial deviation from protocol which we concluded was not warranted. Anecdotally, we can report that certain clinical topics seemed well represented, such as spinal cord injury, physical activity, and chronic pain management.

As with most new concepts, tools, or approaches, it appears that BAP is following a steady trend of uptake over time, with few articles addressing BAP during the first decade after its creation (2002–2012), and most articles addressing BAP appearing during the second decade (2012–2022). There does appear to be a dip in BAP's uptake in the literature during the years 2019 and 2020. This could be explained either because of the COVID-19 pandemic, or as a limitation of this review's inability to locate the full-text file of about 10% of articles originally identified as citations from the literature databases. Although the number of articles discussing the application of BAP is low to date for the year 2023, this is namely due to the timing of this review. In fact, even without needing to conduct an updated search, we are aware of several articles on BAP that have been published in the interim[6] or that are being developed contemporaneously.[16] Thus, we anticipate that the growth of BAP's application in the literature will continue.

That the bulk of articles are from North America is unsurprising, as most of the leading scholars on BAP, including the senior author of this paper, originate from and are currently based in this region. It may be initially surprising that BAP has been applied largely in the community (as compared to clinics or hospitals) and mostly in the context of health care, since generally health care is thought of as taking place within the walls of clinics and hospitals. However, given that BAP was developed to facilitate the self-management support component of the chronic care model for health care transformation, this trend in the literature confirms that BAP is being applied largely in the originally intended place (ie, the community), the intended context (ie, health care), which also aligns with the intended purpose of BAP (ie, an approach to facilitate chronic care via self-management support). That the dominant theoretic frameworks undergirding BAP in the literature is MI, self-management or peer support theory, and various iterations of action planning is further confirmation of the appropriate application of BAP globally.

The relatively unclear or under-reporting of the fidelity of BAP in the literature is a major finding of this scoping review. This finding held true regardless of the domain of fidelity that was examined. This suggests the need for greater dissemination and uptake of formal training methods and programs for students and professionals intending to use BAP in clinical practice or for systems-based change. We suggest this is an area ripe for future research and program evaluation. The authors are aware that some of this work is happening. However, given the rapid uptake of BAP, it may be worthwhile to accelerate specific attention to the measurement and enhancement of fidelity, in order to provide greater guidance on how to ensure that BAP is being taught and applied rigorously and reliably. Given that the fidelity of an intervention often determines its effectiveness in practice, there is an additional strong imperative to accelerate methods to ensure the fidelity of BAP education and application, so that optimal health outcomes can be achieved for the patients and populations for whom BAP is being implemented.

SUMMARY

This scoping review concludes that BAP is being widely disseminated and used with regards to its intended contexts, settings, and theoretic frameworks including in clinical, public health and community practice settings. However, because the fidelity of its application remains unclear or underreported, a high priority for future research should be the exploration of these under-evaluated aspects of BAP. The authors also suggest that greater practical guidance and formal assessment may be necessary for educators, clinicians, and researchers, to support optimal application of BAP in clinical practice or for systems-based change.

CLINICS CARE POINTS

- There is a broad base of evidence currently available about brief action planning (BAP), a pragmatic and motivational interviewing-consistent tool.
- BAP is an approach to health promotion and disease prevention that supports patient self-management, facilitates health behavior change, and enhances health coaching.

- BAP has been applied primarily in North America, within community settings, and evaluated using relatively high-level research designs.
- BAP has mostly been used for health care, and is mostly grounded within the framework of motivational interviewing, as originally intended.
- Although BAP has been applied broadly in health care, the fidelity of BAP remains unclear or underreported, regardless of which fidelity domain is examined.

FUNDING

This project is supported in part by the Health Resources & Services Administration (HRSA) of the US Department of Health & Human Services (HHS) under grant number 1D33HP316710100, Preventive Medicine Residency Training grant, $2000000, 67% financed with nongovernmental sources. This information or content and conclusions are those of the authors and should not be construed as the official position or policy of, nor should any endorsements be inferred by HRSA, HHS, or the US Government. The funder had no role in the conceptualization, design, results, interpretations, or conclusions of the scoping review project described within this article.

DECLARATIONS

None.

CONFLICTS OF INTEREST

There is no conflict of interest in this project.

DISCLOSURE

The authors have no conflicts of interest to disclose.

ACKNOWLEDGMENTS

The authors thank Ms. Wendy Isser, M.L.S., a medical librarian from the Northport VA Medical Center, Northport NY, for her assistance in retrieving the full text of some of the articles identified in this review.

REFERENCES

1. Mathers CD, Boerma T, Ma Fat D. Global and regional causes of death. Br Med Bull 2009;92(1):7–32.
2. Mokdad AH, Marks JS, Stroup DF, et al. Actual causes of death in the United States, 2000. JAMA 2004;291(10):1238–45.
3. Johnson NB, Hayes LD, Brown K, et al. CDC National Health Report: leading causes of morbidity and mortality and associated behavioral risk and protective factors—United States, 2005–2013. 2014.
4. Gutnick D, Reims K, Davis C, et al. Brief Action Planning to Facilitate Behavior Change and Support Patient Self-Management. J Clin Outcome Manag 2014; 21(1):17–29.
5. Cole S, Reims K, Kershner L, et al. Improving care for depression: performance measures, outcomes and insights from the Health Disparities Collaboratives. J Health Care Poor Underserved 2012;23(3):154–73.

6. Cole S, Sannidhi D, Jadotte Y, et al. Using motivational interviewing and brief action planning for adopting and maintaining positive health behaviors. Prog Cardiovasc Dis 2023.

7. Jadotte YT, Lane DS. Population Health Rounds: A Novel Vehicle for Training in Population Medicine and Clinical Preventive Medicine. J Publ Health Manag Pract 2021;27:S139–45.

8. Jadotte YT, Lane DS. Core functions, knowledge bases and essential services: A proposed prescription for the evolution of the preventive medicine specialty. Prev Med 2021;143:106286.

9. Lundahl B, Moleni T, Burke BL, et al. Motivational interviewing in medical care settings: a systematic review and meta-analysis of randomized controlled trials. Patient Educ Counsel 2013;93(2):157–68.

10. Rubak S, Sandbæk A, Lauritzen T, et al. Motivational interviewing: a systematic review and meta-analysis. Br J Gen Pract 2005;55(513):305–12.

11. BAP Professional Network. What is BAP?. Available at: https://bapprofessionalnetwork.org/bap/. Accessed April 21, 2023.

12. Centre for Collaboration Motivation and Innovation. Brief Action Planning. Available at: https://centrecmi.ca/brief-action-planning/. Accessed April 21, 2023.

13. Miller WR, Rollnick S. The effectiveness and ineffectiveness of complex behavioral interventions: impact of treatment fidelity. Contemp Clin Trials 2014;37(2):234–41.

14. Oxford English Dictionary. Fidelity, n. Oxford University Press; 2023.

15. Gearing RE, El-Bassel N, Ghesquiere A, et al. Major ingredients of fidelity: A review and scientific guide to improving quality of intervention research implementation. Clin Psychol Rev 2011;31(1):79–88.

16. Jadotte Y, Cole S. Brief action planning in health and healthcare: a quantitative systematic review protocol. PROSPERO International prospective register of systematic reviews 2023. Available at: https://www.crd.york.ac.uk/prospero/display_record.php?ID=CRD42023397512.

17. Cole S, Bogenschutz M, Hungerford D. Motivational interviewing and psychiatry: Use in addiction treatment, risky drinking and routine practice. Focus 2011;9(1):42–54.

18. Connell G, Verville L, Cancelliere C, et al. Brief action planning targeting prognostic factors for an adult with persistent low back pain without radiculopathy: A case report. Clinical case reports 2020;8(12):2776–80.

19. Farmer AJ, Oke J, Hardeman W, et al. The effect of a brief action planning intervention on adherence to double-blind study medication, compared to a standard trial protocol, in the Atorvastatin in Factorial with Omega EE90 Risk Reduction in Diabetes (AFORRD) clinical trial: A cluster randomised sub-study. Diabetes Res Clin Pract 2016;120:56–64.

20. Worley P. Open thinking, closed questioning: Two kinds of open and closed question. Journal of Philosophy in Schools 2015;2(2):17–29.

21. Peters MD, Godfrey CM, Khalil H, et al. Guidance for conducting systematic scoping reviews. Int J Evid Base Healthc 2015. https://doi.org/10.1097/xeb.0000000000000050.

22. Peters MD, Marnie C, Tricco AC, et al. Updated methodological guidance for the conduct of scoping reviews. JBI evidence synthesis 2020;18(10):2119–26.

23. Jadotte YT. Brief Action Planning in Health and Healthcare: A Scoping Review Protocol. 2023. https://doi.org/10.17605/OSF.IO/AT4VE

24. McGowan J, Straus S, Moher D, et al. Reporting scoping reviews—PRISMA ScR extension. Journal of clinical epidemiology 2020;123:177–9.

25. Tricco AC, Lillie E, Zarin W, et al. PRISMA extension for scoping reviews (PRISMA-ScR): checklist and explanation. Annals of internal medicine 2018; 169(7):467–73.

26. Snilstveit B, Vojtkova M, Bhavsar A, et al. Evidence & Gap Maps: A tool for promoting evidence informed policy and strategic research agendas. Journal of clinical epidemiology 2016;79:120–9.

APPENDIX 1: SEARCH STRATEGY

Databases (Platform) or Registers	Search Date	Search Terms	Number of Articles
Medline (Ovid)	March 1, 2023	("brief action planning" OR "brief action plan").mp. [mp = title, book title, abstract, original title, name of substance word, subject heading word, floating sub-heading word, keyword heading word, organism supplementary concept word, protocol supplementary concept word, rare disease supplementary concept word, unique identifier, synonyms]	13
CINAHL Plus (EBSCOhost)	March 1, 2023	"brief action planning" OR "brief action plan"	15
ScienceDirect	March 1, 2023	"brief action planning" OR "brief action plan"	42
PsycInfo (EBSCOhost)	March 1, 2023	"brief action planning" OR "brief action plan"	2
Google Scholar	March 1, 2023	"brief action planning"	280
Web of Science	March 1, 2023	(ALL=("brief action planning")) OR ALL=("brief action plan")	17
Academic Search Complete (EBSCOhost)	March 1, 2023	"brief action planning" OR "brief action plan"	7
Clinicaltrials.gov	March 1, 2023	"brief action planning" OR "brief action plan"	1
Cochrane Library	March 1, 2023	"brief action planning" OR "brief action plan"	20

(continued on next page)

(continued)

Databases (Platform) or Registers	Search Date	Search Terms	Number of Articles
ProQuest	March 1, 2023	"brief action planning" OR "brief action plan"	96
PubMed	March 1, 2023	"brief action planning" OR "brief action plan"	13
WHO ICTRP	March 1, 2023	"brief action planning" OR "brief action plan"	2
TOTAL CITATIONS FROM DATABASES AND REGISTERS			508
Organization Websites	Search Date	Search Terms	Number of articles
American Psychological Association	March 15, 2023	"brief action planning"	0
American Psychiatric Association (APA)	March 15, 2023	"brief action planning"	0
Association of Consultation Liaison Psychiatrists (ACLP)	March 15, 2023	"brief action planning"	0
American College of Physicians (ACP)	March 15, 2023	"brief action planning"	0
New York Chapter of the American College of Physicians (NY ACP)	March 15, 2023	"brief action planning"	2
Motivational Interviewing Network of Trainers (MINT)	March 15, 2023	"brief action planning"	30
Institute for Healthcare Improvement (IHI)	March 15, 2023	"brief action planning"	4
Substance Abuse and Mental Health Services Administration (SAMHSA)	March 15, 2023	"brief action planning"	0
Health Resources and Services Administration (HRSA)	March 15, 2023	"brief action planning"	0
Centers for Disease Control and Prevention (CDC)	March 15, 2023	"brief action planning"	0
Indian Health Service (HIS)	March 15, 2023	"brief action planning"	1
Citation Chasing and Hand Searching	March 15, 2023	N/A	5
TOTAL CITATIONS FROM OTHER SOURCES			42

APPENDIX 2: DATA EXTRACTION INSTRUMENT

Evidence Source Details and Characteristics	
Citation details (eg, author/s, date, title, journal, volume, issue, pages)	
Country/Region	
Context (eg, community, hospital, clinic, school)	
Types of evidence source (eg, study design)	
Participants (details eg, age/sex and number)	
Details/Results Extracted from Source of Evidence (in Relation to the Concept of the ScR)	
Context of BAP application (eg, health, healthcare, education, business)	
Assessment of BAP fidelity in clinical care delivery or systems implementation: design, training, monitoring intervention delivery, and monitoring intervention receipt (eg, whether all 8 competencies were taught, whether any elements of the BAP algorithm were modified, or whether MI was integrated into BAP or vice versa and how this was accomplished)	Design Training Monitoring intervention delivery Monitoring intervention receipt Other aspect of fidelity
Discipline or profession where BAP was used (eg, mental health, psychiatry, community health, nursing)	
Conceptual or theoretic grounding of BAP	

APPENDIX 3: LIST OF STUDIES EXCLUDED VIA FULL-TEXT REVIEW WITH REASONS FOR EXCLUSION

Databases and Registers.

(2011). "Motivate change: Use a few key questions." *Patient Education Management* 18(4): 41 to 43.

- Not available.

(2013). Active Lives: Transforming Ourselves and Our Patients, Part 3. *Academic Video Online*, Healthy Learning.

- Not available.

(2017). "Brief Action Planning (BAP): A Self-Management Support Technique for Promoting Collaborative Goal Setting for Patients on Home Dialysis." *AMERICAN JOURNAL OF KIDNEY DISEASES* 69(4): A64.

- Not available.

(2017). "Dialysis Prescription, Sun Exposure and Vitamin D Levels in Hispanic Patients on Hemodialysis." *AMERICAN JOURNAL OF KIDNEY DISEASES* 69(4): A64.

- Not available.

Adamo, K., et al. "Desi-GDM Trial Protocol Version 6.0 A culturally-tailored personalizeD nutrition intErvention in South ASIan women at risk of Gestational Diabetes Mellitus (DESI-GDM)–a randomized trial Principal Investigator: Russell de Souza, ScD, RD."

- Not available.

Ahuja, T. K., et al. (2022). "Teaching Second-Year Medical Students How to Counsel Pediatric Patients with Unhealthy Body Mass Index." *Childhood Obesity*.

- Not available.

Akhter, K., et al. (2022). "A Systematic Review and Meta-analysis of Face-to-face Medication Adherence Interventions for Patients with Long Term Health Conditions." *ANNALS OF BEHAVIORAL MEDICINE* 56(12): 1218 to 1230.

- Wrong concept (not BAP or its application).

Albelbisi, Z. (2021). The Effectiveness of Information-Motivation-Behavioural Skills Model-Based Diabetes Self-Management Education Among Patients with Type 2 Diabetes (Imbdsme): Randomized Clinical Trial. England, The University of Nottingham (United Kingdom).

- Not available.

Bickley, L. and P. G. Szilagyi (2012). *Bates' guide to physical examination and history-taking*, Lippincott Williams & Wilkins.

- Wrong concept (not BAP or its application).

Bigand, T. L. (2019). "1E. 3. Risk for Overeating to Cope with Pain among Obese Adults with Chronic Pain." *PAIN MANAGEMENT NURSING* 20(2): 95.

- Wrong concept (not BAP or its application).

Brady, T. J. (2016). "Enhancing Clinical Practice with Community-Based Self-Management Support Programs." *Psychosocial Factors in Arthritis: Perspectives on Adjustment and Management*: 255 to 272.

- Wrong concept (not BAP or its application).

Brooks, A. J., et al. (2020). "Introducing integrative primary health care to an interprofessional audience: Feasibility and impact of an asynchronous online course." *EXPLORE* 16(6): 392 to 400.

- Wrong concept (not BAP or its application).

Brooks, A. J., et al. (2021). "Professional development in integrative health through an interprofessional online course in clinical settings." *EXPLORE* 17(6): 505 to 512.

- Wrong concept (not BAP or its application).

Bussières, A. (2017). "Canadian Chiropractic Guideline Initiative (CCGI) progress and future directions: December 2017." *The Journal of the Canadian Chiropractic Association* 61(3): 186.

- Wrong concept (not BAP or its application).

Bussières, A. E., et al. (2015). "Fast tracking the design of theory-based KT interventions through a consensus process." *IMPLEMENTATION SCIENCE* 10(1): 1 to 14.

- Wrong concept (not BAP or its application).

Bussières, A. E., et al. (2016). "The Treatment of Neck Pain–Associated Disorders and Whiplash-Associated Disorders: A Clinical Practice Guideline." *Journal of Manipulative and Physiologic Therapeutics* 39(8): 523 to 564.e527.

- Wrong concept (not BAP or its application).

Cadel, L., et al. (2020). "Exploring the perspectives on medication self-management among persons with spinal cord injury/dysfunction and providers." *Research in Social and Administrative Pharmacy* 16(12): 1775 to 1784.

- Wrong concept (not BAP or its application).

CARVLIN, A. and M. ELSNER "Piloting a Coordinated System of Care for Childhood Obesity." *IllinoisPediatrician*: 6.

- Wrong concept (not BAP or its application).

Chemtob, K., et al. (2018). "Exploring the peer mentorship experiences of adults with spinal cord injury." *Rehabilitation psychology* 63(4): 542.

- Wrong concept (not BAP or its application).

Christison, A. L. (2015). *Pediatric Obesity Prevention in Primary Care: Employing Brief Action Planning with Obesigenic Behavior Screening*. 2015 AAP National Conference and Exhibition, American Academy of Pediatrics.

- Wrong concept (not BAP or its application).

Chung, H., et al. (2019). "Evaluation of a Continuum-Based Behavioral Health Integration Framework Among Small Primary Care Practices in New York State: Practice and Policy Findings and Recommendations." *United Hospital Fund and New York State Health Foundation*.

- Wrong concept (not BAP or its application).

Clark, W. (2013). "Risky Drinking and Interviewing About Alcohol Use." *The Medical Interview E-Book: The Three Function Approach*: 243.

- Wrong concept (not BAP or its application).

Clayton, C. (2016). A pilot randomized trial of a novel intervention to promote physical activity in people with knee osteoarthritis: protocol and baseline analysis from the TRACK-OA study, University of British Columbia.

- Wrong concept (not BAP or its application).

Cole, S., et al. (2013). "Function three: collaborate for management." *The Medical Interview E-Book: The Three Function Approach*: 34.

- Duplicate report.

Cole, S., et al. (2014). "Brief action planning: a self-management support and motivational interviewing technique for the routine practice of medicine, psychiatry, and disease management." *Psychosomatic Medicine* 76(3): A46-A47.

- Not available.

Cole, S., et al. (2013). "Stepped-care advanced skills for action planning." *The Medical Interview E-Book: The Three Function Approach*: 125.

- Duplicate report.

Cole, S. A. and J. Bird (2013). *The medical interview e-book: The three function approach*, Elsevier Health Sciences.

- Duplicate report.

Cradock, K. A., et al. (2022). "Design of a Planner-Based Intervention to Facilitate Diet Behavior Change in Type 2 Diabetes." *Sensors* 22(7): 2795.

- Wrong concept (not BAP or its application).

Cranston, K. (2019). Sustainability of motivational interviewing skills in new Small Steps for Big Changes coaches, University of British Columbia.

- Wrong concept (not BAP or its application).

Davis, A. (2017). Camp-Based Intervention for Overweight Children with Developmental Disabilities. United States—California, Loma Linda University: 81.

- Wrong concept (not BAP or its application).

Davis, C. (2014). "The Brief Action Planning Guide-A Self–Management Support Tool for Chronic Conditions, Health and Wellness."

- Not available.

Davis, C. and S. Cole (2013). "Communicating with Patients with Chronic Illness." *The Medical Interview E-Book: The Three Function Approach*: 145.

- Wrong concept (not BAP or its application).

DeShaw, K. J. (2019). Methods and Evaluation of a Health Coach Training Practicum Experience for Healthy Lifestyle Behavior Change. United States–Iowa, Iowa State University: 172.

- Wrong concept (not BAP or its application).

Dhopte, P. (2016). Chiropractors Can Do: Testing the Feasibility of Intervening to Optimize Chiropractic Care for Adults with Neck Pain Disorders: A Pilot Cluster Randomized Controlled Trial. Canada–Quebec, CA, McGill University (Canada): 117.

- Duplicate report.

Dhopte, P., et al. (2016). "Testing the feasibility of a knowledge translation intervention designed to improve chiropractic care for adults with neck pain disorders: study protocol for a pilot cluster-randomized controlled trial." *Pilot Feasibility Stud* 2: 33.
- Duplicate report.

Domke, A. (2022). Insights into the Mechanisms of Action Planning Interventions in the Context of Fruit and Vegetable Consumption.
- Wrong concept (not BAP or its application).

Domke, A., et al. (2021). "Immediate effects of a very brief planning intervention on fruit and vegetable consumption: a randomized controlled trial." *Applied Psychology: Health and Well-Being* 13(2): 377 to 393.
- Wrong concept (not BAP or its application).

Domke, A., et al. (2022). "Plan pursuit in the context of daily fruit and vegetable consumption: The importance of cue detection and the execution of the planned behavior for overall behavior change." British Journal of Health Psychology 27(3): 1172 to 1187.
- Wrong concept (not BAP or its application).

Dorstyn, D., et al. (2019). "Can targeted job-information for adults with spinal cord dysfunction be effectively delivered online? A pilot study." *The journal of spinal cord medicine* 42(1): 94 to 101.
- Wrong concept (not BAP or its application).

Duncan-Carnesciali, J. (2016). An evaluation of the innovation of e-health featuring a diabetes self-management program delivered using avatar-based technology: Findings with certified diabetes educators and adults living with type 2 diabetes mellitis. United States–New York, Teachers College, Columbia University: 250.
- Wrong concept (not BAP or its application).

Duong, M. T., et al. (2016). "Twelve-Month Outcomes of a Randomized Trial of the Positive Thoughts and Action Program for Depression Among Early Adolescents." *Prevention Science* 17(3): 295 to 305.
- Not available.

Eilayyan, O., et al. (2022). "Promoting the use of a self-management strategy among novice chiropractors treating individuals with spine pain: A mixed methods pilot clustered-clinical trial." PLoS One 17(1).
- Wrong concept (not BAP or its application).

Elmaci, O. (2014). "A model proposal concerning balance scorecard (bsc) application integratedwith resource consumption accounting (rca) in enterprise performance management." International Journal of Organizational Leadership 3(1): 1 to 9.
- Not available.

Erder, M. and P. Pureur (2016). Chapter 6-Validating the Architecture. Continuous Architecture. M. Erder and P. Pureur. Boston, Morgan Kaufmann: 131 to 159.
- Not available.

ES, B. "Bates. Guia de exploracion fisica 12ª edicion."
- Not available.

Falck, R. S., et al. (2020). "Effect of a multimodal lifestyle intervention on sleep and cognitive function in older adults with probable mild cognitive impairment and poor sleep: a randomized clinical trial." *Journal of Alzheimer's Disease* 76(1): 179 to 193.
- Wrong concept (not BAP or its application).

Farnier, M., et al. (2017). "Long-term treatment adherence to the proprotein convertase subtilisin/kexin type 9 inhibitor alirocumab in 6 ODYSSEY Phase III clinical studies with treatment duration of 1 to 2 years." *Journal of clinical lipidology* 11(4): 986 to 997.
- Wrong concept (not BAP or its application).

Flood, S. M. (2018). Determining the Impact of an Educational Intervention on Family Medicine Residents' Social Cognitions and Behavior for Discussing Physical Activity. Canada–Ontario, CA, Queen's University (Canada): 198.
- Wrong concept (not BAP or its application).

Flood, S. M., et al. (2019). "Prescription exercise at Queen's: A prospective program evaluation of physical activity effects among university students with depression and anxiety." *Journal of Exercise, Movement, and Sport (SCAPPS refereed abstracts repository)* 51(1): 199 to 199.
- Not available.

Fukumori, R. H. (2016). The Motley Tower: Master Plans, Urban Crises, and Multiracial Higher Education in Postwar Los Angeles. United States–California, University of Southern California: 438.
- Not available.

Gainforth, H. L., et al. (2014). *Testing the feasibility of training peers with spinal cord injury (SCI) to learn and implement brief action planning to promote physical activity to people with SCI.* ANNALS OF BEHAVIORAL MEDICINE, SPRINGER 233 SPRING ST, NEW YORK, NY 10013 USA.
- Duplicate report.

Gainforth, H. L., et al. (2019). "Investigating characteristics of quality peer mentors with spinal cord injury." *ARCHIVES OF PHYSICAL MEDICINE AND REHABILITATION* 100(10): 1916 to 1923.
- Wrong concept (not BAP or its application).

Gainforth, H. L., et al. (2015). "Testing the feasibility of training peers with a spinal cord injury to learn and implement brief action planning to promote physical activity to people with spinal cord injury." *JOURNAL OF SPINAL CORD MEDICINE* 38(4): 515 to 525.
- Duplicate report.

Gainforth, H. L., et al. (2015). "Using network analysis to understand knowledge mobilization in a community-based organization." *International Journal of Behavioral Medicine* 22: 292 to 300.
- Wrong concept (not BAP or its application).

Gassaway, J., et al. (2017). "Effects of peer mentoring on self-efficacy and hospital readmission after inpatient rehabilitation of individuals with spinal cord injury: a randomized controlled trial." *ARCHIVES OF PHYSICAL MEDICINE AND REHABILITATION* 98(8): 1526 to 1534. e1522.
- Wrong concept (not BAP or its application).

Gierc, M. S. H. (2021). Development and Initial Testing of a Brief Mindfulness Meditation Training Intervention for Preoperative Patients: An Application of the Orbit Model. Canada–Ontario, CA, Queen's University (Canada): 459.
- Wrong concept (not BAP or its application).

Huang, Y. (2020). Internet of Things enabled sedentary behavior change in office workers: development and feasibility of a novel intervention (WorkMyWay), University of Nottingham.
- Duplicate report.

Isrctn (2021). "Promoting the use of a self-management intervention among chiropractic students treating individuals with back pain." https://trialsearch.who.int/Trial2.aspx?TrialID = ISRCTN17077842.
- Wrong concept (not BAP or its application).

Johnson, A. M. (2021). A Descriptive Study Exploring the Components of Academic Coaching Programs in Nursing Education Across the Midwest. United States–Nebraska, Bryan College of Health Sciences: 91.

- Wrong context (not health or healthcare).

Kasidi, J. (2022). "Quality Improvement Project Utilizing a Comprehensive Toolkit with Individualized Food Label Education and Brief Action Planning for Healthy Food Choices to Reduce the Burden of Chronic Disease Among Black People in the United States." *NURSING RESEARCH* 71(3): S104-S104.
- Wrong concept (not BAP or its application).

Larié, S. (2019). Provider Evaluation of a Lower Carbohydrate Nutrition Education Video for People with Type 1 and Type 2 Diabetes. United States–Arizona, The University of Arizona: 92.
- Wrong concept (not BAP or its application).

Leese, J., et al. (2021). "Experiences of wearable technology by persons with knee osteoarthritis participating in a physical activity counseling intervention study: a relational ethics lens." *Arthritis & rheumatology* 73(SUPPL 9): 2228 to 2229.
- Duplicate report.

Magasi, S. and C. Papadimitriou (2022). "Peer support interventions in physical medicine and rehabilitation: a framework to advance the field." *Archives Of Physical Medicine And Rehabilitation* 103(7): S222-S229.
- Wrong concept (not BAP or its application).

McIntosh, C. A. (2017). A mixed methods study of the motivational influences upon dietitian change of counseling practice, Nipissing University, Faculty of Education.
- Wrong concept (not BAP or its application).

McKay, R. C., et al. (2022). "Investigating the peer Mentor-Mentee relationship: characterizing peer mentorship conversations between people with spinal cord injury." *Disability and Rehabilitation*: 1 to 12.
- Wrong concept (not BAP or its application).

McNamara, M. and T. Bodenheimer (2019). "Training medical students in health coaching skills." *MedEdPublish* 8(106): 106.
- Wrong concept (not BAP or its application).

Med, T. B. (2014). "Ploughman and colleagues" *Implement Sci* 9: 30.
- Not available.

Mendoza, M. A. (2017). Teaching and motivating patients to achieve treatment goals. *Principles of Diabetes Mellitus: Third Edition*, Springer International Publishing: 823 to 842.
- Not available.

Miano, a. And e. Wegner "elise butkiewicz, antonia carbone, stuart green." *The Behavioral Health Specialist in Primary Care*: 73.
- Not available.

Mihalko, S. L., et al. (2023). Chapter 4-Core components of best evidence OA care: management planning, education, supporting self-management and behavior change. *Osteoarthritis Health Professional Training Manual*. D. J. Hunter and J. P. Eyles, Academic Press: 55 to 72.
- Not available.

Mikrut, C. L. (2022). Comparing the Effects of an Adjunct Brief Action Planning Intervention to Standard Treatment in a Heterogeneous Sample of Chronic Pain Patients. United States–Illinois, Illinois Institute of Technology: 103.
- Not available.

Milligan, J., et al. (2019). "Primary care perspective in managing sexual health for individuals with spinal cord injuries–Development of educational material for primary care providers." *The journal of spinal cord medicine* 42(S1): S242.
- Not available.

Mitchell, E. G., et al. (2020). *Characterizing Human vs. Automated Coaching: Preliminary Results*. Extended Abstracts of the 2020 CHI Conference on Human Factors in Computing Systems.
- Not available.
Moore, P. and F. Cole (2008). "The pain toolkit." *London, UK: NHS.*
- Wrong concept (not BAP or its application).
Munro, S., et al. (2020). "Decision-Making Needs, Challenges, and Opportunities Among Health Care Professionals Supporting Infant Feeding Choices: A Qualitative Investigation Involving Expert Interviews." *MEDICAL DECISION MAKING* 40(1): E16-E17.
- Wrong concept (not BAP or its application).
Muskin, P. R., et al. (2019). *Study Guide to Consultation-Liaison Psychiatry: A Companion to The American Psychiatric Association Publishing Textbook of Psychosomatic Medicine and Consultation-Liaison Psychiatry*, American Psychiatric Pub.
- Not available.
Nct (2014). "Reducing Distress And Improving Glycemic Control In Adults With Type 1 Diabetes." https://clinicaltrials.gov/show/NCT02175732.
- Wrong concept (not BAP or its application).
Nct (2022). "Improving Comprehensive Care of Cancer Patients." https://clinicaltrials.gov/show/NCT05323409.
- Wrong concept (not BAP or its application).
Nover, C. H. (2013). Effective primary care for individuals with serious mental illness: An intervention and systematic review. United States–Utah, The University of Utah: 112.
- Wrong concept (not BAP or its application).
O'Shaughnessy, D. F. and M. Tilki (2007). "Cultural competency in physiotherapy: a model for training." *Physiotherapy* 93(1): 69 to 77.
- Wrong concept (not BAP or its application).
Olivieri, C. "Short Term Intervention Using the Paleolithic Diet to Prevent Progression from Prediabetes to Type 2 Diabetes in Those with HgA1c 5.7% or Higher."
- Wrong concept (not BAP or its application).
Orbell, S. and L. Alison Phillips (2019). "Automatic processes and self-regulation of illness." *Health Psychology Review* 13(4): 378 to 405.
- Wrong concept (not BAP or its application).
Ovbiagbonhia, A. R. (2021). Learning to Innovate: How to Foster Innovation Competence in Students of Built Environment at Universities of Applied Sciences. Netherlands, Wageningen University and Research: 227.
- Wrong context (not health or healthcare).
Patel, M. L. (2018). Comparing Self-monitoring Strategies for Weight Loss: Does Developing Mastery Before Diet Tracking Enhance Engagement? United States–North Carolina, Duke University: 222.
- Wrong concept (not BAP or its application).
Pearlman, R. E. and C. Chou (2019). "Communication Skills Training to Enhance Patient Adherence." *Psychiatric Nonadherence: A Solutions-Based Approach*: 103 to 112.
- Not available.
Perrier, M.-J. and K. A. M. Ginis (2017). Communicating physical activity information to people with physical disabilities. *Persuasion and communication in sport, exercise, and physical activity*, Routledge: 233 to 249.
- Not available.

Pierce, J. D. (2015). Alliance-building strategies as a critical component of coaching: Effects of feedback and analysis on coach practice, teacher practice, and alliance. United States–Washington, University of Washington: 153.
- Wrong context (not health or healthcare).

Pomarensky, M., et al. (2022). "Management of Chronic Musculoskeletal Pain Through a Biopsychosocial Lens." *Journal of Athletic Training* 57(4): 312 to 318.
- Duplicate report.

Puatu, S. S. (2020). The Effects of Small Changes Approach in Combination with Motivational Interviewing on Behavioral Weight Loss Management among Overweight and Obese Adult Women. United States–California, Brandman University: 71.
- Wrong concept (not BAP or its application).

Pyle, S. "Updated: Motivational Interviewing: The One Tool Every Behavioral Health Provider Needs UPDATED: Motivational Interviewing: The One Tool Every Behavioral Health Provider Needs."
- Wrong concept (not BAP or its application).

Rai, R. K. (2004). Development and implementation of technology plans in Tennessee public school systems. United States–Tennessee, The University of Tennessee: 207.
- Wrong context (not health or healthcare).

Reyes Fernández, B. (2015). Social Support, Planning and Action Control in Self-Regulatory Health Behavior Processes.
- Wrong concept (not BAP or its application).

Reyes Fernández, B., et al. "A brief action planning intervention increases physical exercise among less active young adults." *Social Support, Planning and Action Control in Self-Regulatory Health Behavior Processes*: 97.
- Duplicate report.

Reyes, H. L. M., et al. (2022). "Web-Based Delivery of a Family-Based Dating Violence Prevention Program for Youth Who Have Been Exposed to Intimate Partner Violence: Protocol for an Acceptability and Feasibility Study." *JMIR Research Protocols* 11(8).
- Wrong concept (not BAP or its application).

Reyneke, R., et al. "The use of implementation theories, models, and frameworks in veterinary medicine–protocol for a scoping review."
- Wrong population (not adults or children).

Ryan, P., et al. (2020). "Self-management processes used by healthy middle-aged women to change behaviors." *Western Journal of Nursing Research* 42(5): 321 to 331.
- Wrong concept (not BAP or its application).

Schedule, D. "Advanced Motivational Interviewing."
- Wrong concept (not BAP or its application).

Schwartz, M. D., et al. (2014). "The use of panel management assistants to improve smoking cessation and hypertension management by VA primary care teams: a cluster randomized controlled trial." *Journal of general internal medicine* 29: S234-S235.
- Duplicate.

Shah, A., et al. (2015). "Protect your heart: a culture-specific multimedia cardiovascular health education program." *Journal of health communication* 20(4): 424 to 430.
- Wrong concept (not BAP or its application).

Shimazaki, T., et al. (2022). "The process of behavioral change in individuals who are uninterested in health: a qualitative study based on professional health knowledge." *Environmental Health and Preventive Medicine* 27: 32 to 32.
- Wrong concept (not BAP or its application).

Shleyaust, A. and N. L. CRAIG (2019). "Transgender Affirmative COgnitive-Behavioral Therapy." *Handbook of Evidence-Based Mental Health Practice with Sexual and Gender Minorities*: 74.
- Wrong concept (not BAP or its application).

Singh, H. (2020). Understanding the Complexity of Falls and Fall Prevention for Wheelchair Users with Spinal Cord Injury Across the Continuum of Care. Canada–Ontario, CA, University of Toronto (Canada): 172.
- Wrong concept (not BAP or its application).

Singh, H., et al. (2020). "Perspectives of wheelchair users with spinal cord injury on fall circumstances and fall prevention: A mixed methods approach using photovoice." *PLoS One* 15(8).
- Wrong concept (not BAP or its application).

Singh, H., et al. (2020). "Factors that influence the risk of falling after spinal cord injury: a qualitative photo-elicitation study with individuals that use a wheelchair as their primary means of mobility." *BMJ Open* 10(2).
- Wrong concept (not BAP or its application).

Smith, P., et al. (2018). "Feasibility and acceptability of a cancer symptom awareness intervention for adults living in socioeconomically deprived communities." *BMC Public Health* 18.
- Wrong concept (not BAP or its application).

Sniehotta, F. F., et al. (2007). "Randomized controlled trial of a one-minute intervention changing oral self-care behavior." *Journal of Dental Research* 86(7): 641 to 645.
- Wrong concept (not BAP or its application).

Squires, A. (2014). "English ability and glycemic control in Latinos with diabetes." *J. Clin. Outcomes Manag* 21: 299 to 301.

Stern, M., et al. (2021). "A cluster-randomized control trial targeting parents of pediatric cancer survivors with obesity: Rationale and study protocol of Nourish-T+." *Contemporary Clinical Trials* 102: 106,296.
- Wrong concept (not BAP or its application).

Swanson, M. (2016). "Implementation of an SMART Goal Intervention for Diabetic Patients: A Practice Change in Primary Care."
- Wrong concept (not BAP or its application).

Sweet, S. N., et al. (2018). "Spinal cord injury peer mentorship: applying self-determination theory to explain quality of life and participation." *Archives Of Physical Medicine And Rehabilitation* 99(3): 468 to 476. e412.
- Wrong concept (not BAP or its application).

Tumpa, J., et al. (2020). "The development of electronic brief action planning (e-bap): a self-management support tool for health behavior change." *Medical Decision Making* 40(1): E216-E216.
- Duplicate report.

Unsworth, J., et al. (2016). "Improving performance amongst nursing students through the discovery of discrepancies during simulation." *Nurse Education in Practice* 16(1): 47 to 53.
- Wrong concept (not BAP or its application).

Vaughn, L. M., et al. (2019). "Developing and implementing a stress and coping intervention in partnership with Latino immigrant coresearchers." *Translational Issues in Psychological Science* 5(1): 62.
- Wrong concept (not BAP or its application).

Villegas Rodriguez, N. A. (2012). Developing and piloting an internet based STI and HIV prevention intervention among young Chilean women. United States–Florida, University of Miami: 371.

- Wrong concept (not BAP or its application).

Viner, J., et al. "An Exploration of "Forgiveness" in a Clinical Population of Emerging Adults David Daskovsky, PhD "Minding The Brain": A Developmental Neurobiological Model for Substance Abuse Treatment in Emerging Adults."
- Duplicate report.

Wolff, M. M. (2018). Facilitating Lifestyle Behavior Change in the Primary Care Setting with a Staged Approach to Childhood Obesity Treatment. United States–Iowa, Iowa State University: 171.
- Duplicate report.

Yan, J., et al. (2014). "The effect of a telephone follow-up intervention on illness perception and lifestyle after myocardial Infarction in China: A randomized controlled trial." *International Journal of Nursing Studies* 51(6): 844 to 855.
- Wrong concept (not BAP or its application).

Yang, M. C., et al. (2022). "Preliminary investigation of the student-delivered Community Outreach teleheAlth program for Covid education and Health promotion (COACH)." *Family Practice*.
- Duplicate report.

Zhao, Z. and X. Wang (2019). "Application of Multidisciplinary Intervention Model in Nursing of Older patients with Diabetes."
- Wrong concept (not BAP or its application).

Other Sources.

Cole, S. (2011). *Seeking Research Collaborators to evaluate Online Learning Application of MI- "Brief Action Planning*. Retrieved March 15 from https://motivationalinterviewing.org/forum/seeking-research-collaborators-evaluate-online-learning-application-mi-brief-action-planning.
- Wrong concept (no application of BAP).

Cole, S. (2020). *Brief Action Planning and Current Status of MI-request update help*. Retrieved March 15 from https://motivationalinterviewing.org/forum/brief-action-planning-and-current-status-mi-request-update-help.
- Wrong concept (not BAP or its application).

Cole, S. (2020). *MI for Emerging Era of Telemedicine-request for references, slide sets, ideas*. Retrieved March 15 from https://motivationalinterviewing.org/forum/mi-emerging-era-telemedicine-request-references-slide-sets-ideas.
- Wrong concept (not BAP or its application).

Davis, C. (2017). *What Is Motivational Interviewing?* Institute for Healthcare Improvement. Retrieved March 15 from https://www.ihi.org/education/IHIOpenSchool/resources/Pages/AudioandVideo/ConnieDavis-WhatIsMotivationalInterviewing.aspx.
- Wrong concept (not BAP or its application).

Davis, C. (2017). *What Is "Ask, Tell, Ask"?* Institute for Healthcare Improvement. Retrieved March 15 from https://www.ihi.org/education/IHIOpenSchool/resources/Pages/AudioandVideo/ConnieDavis-WhatIsAskTellAsk.aspx.
- Wrong concept (not BAP or its application).

Davis, C. (2017). *What Is Teach-Back?* Institute for Healthcare Improvement. Retrieved March 15 from https://www.ihi.org/education/IHIOpenSchool/resources/Pages/AudioandVideo/ConnieDavis-WhatIsTeachBack.aspx.
- Wrong concept (not BAP or its application).

APPENDIX 4: CHARACTERISTICS OF INCLUDED STUDIES

Citation (Author-Title) Year	Country or Region	Context (ie, Site of Participants)	Types of Evidence Source (eg, Study Design)	Context of BAP Application	Discipline or Profession of BAP Use	Conceptual or Theoretic Grounding of BAP (Type)
Allin et al, 2019	Canada	Community	Mixed Methods	Healthcare	Peer Specialists	Motivational Interviewing
Allin et al, 2020	Canada	Community	Mixed Methods	Health	Health Coaching	Motivational Interviewing
American Psychiatric Association 2022	USA	N/A	Online Course or Workshop	Healthcare	Psychiatry	Motivational Interviewing
Applegate et al, 2021	USA	Clinic	Randomized Control Trial	Healthcare	Nursing; Health Coaching	Action Planning Theory
Ayyoub et al, 2017	UK	Community	Pre and post test	Health	Kinesiology; Community Health	Health Action Process Approach; Self-Efficacy Theory
Brathwaite et al, 2018	USA	Community	Pilot study	Healthcare	Nursing; Geriatric	Motivational Interviewing
Brody et al, 2015	USA	Community	Pilot study	Healthcare	Peer Specialists	Peer Health Coach Model; Transtheoretical Model; Social Cognitive Theory
Bruckenthal 2019	USA	School	Educational Session	Education	Nursing; Pain Medicine	Motivational Interviewing
Clayton et al, 2015	Canada	Community	Feasibility study	Healthcare	Physical Therapy	Motivational Interviewing
Cole 2012	International	School	Online video	Healthcare	Primary Care	Motivational Interviewing

(continued on next page)

(continued)

Citation (Author-Title) Year	Country or Region	Context (ie, Site of Participants)	Types of Evidence Source (eg, Study Design)	Context of BAP Application	Discipline or Profession of BAP Use	Conceptual or Theoretic Grounding of BAP (Type)
Cole 2011	USA	N/A	Clinical synthesis	Education	Psychiatry	Motivational Interviewing
Cole et al, 2021	USA	School	Survey	Healthcare	Preventive Medicine; Psychiatry	Motivational Interviewing
Cole-Function Three 2013	USA	N/A	Book Chapter	Healthcare	Medical Education	Motivational Interviewing
Cole-Stepped Care 2013	USA	N/A	Textbook	Education	Medical Education	Motivational Interviewing
Connell et al, 2020	Canada	Community	Case Report	Healthcare	Chiropractor	Brief-Action Planning
Davis 2012	USA	N/A	Lecture	Healthcare		
Davis 2017	USA	School	Online Video	Healthcare	General Medicine	
Deegala & Champany, 2017	USA	School	Course	Healthcare	Dentistry	Motivational Interviewing
Dhopte et al, 2019	Canada	Clinic	Pilot Clustered Randomized Control Trial	Healthcare	Chiropractor	Motivational Interviewing
Duncan et al, 2018	USA	Community	Cross-section study with quantitative and qualitative paradigms	Healthcare	Nursing; Community Health Educator	
Eilayyan 2017	Canada	Clinic	Knowledge Translation Intervention	Healthcare	Primary Care; Nursing; Psychology; Physical Therapy	Brief-Action Planning

Study	Country	Setting	Study design	Sector	Provider	Theory
Eilayyan et al, 2018	Canada	School	Mixed methods design	Self-management support education	Chiropractor	Motivational Interviewing
Eilayyan et al, 2019	Canada	School	Prospective cohort study	Healthcare	Chiropractor	Motivational Interviewing
Falck et al, 2020	Canada	N/A	Systemic review of observation studies, randomized control trial	Healthcare	Physical Therapy	Motivational Interviewing
Falck-Buying-Time 2018	Canada	Community	Randomized control trial	Healthcare	Geriatric	
Falck-Can-We-Improve 2018	Canada	Community	Randomized control trial	Healthcare	Physical Therapy	Motivational Interviewing
Farmer et al, 2016	UK	Clinic, community	Two-arm adherence study within randomized control drug trial	Healthcare	Primary Care	
Gainforth, 2013	Canada	Clinic	Single group pre-post design	Health	Peer Specialists	Motivational Interviewing; Theory of Planned Behavior
Galaviz et al, 2018	USA	N/A	Systematic review	Healthcare	Lifestyle Medicine	
Gallegos-Carrillo et al, 2016	Mexico	Clinic	Cluster randomized trial	Healthcare	Primary Care	
Gaughan & 2017	USA	Community	Community intervention-design not specified	Health	Community Health Educators	
Gaughan & Brinckman, 2018	USA	Community	Prospective cohort study	Education	Community Health Educators	Motivational Interviewing

(continued on next page)

(continued)

Citation (Author-Title) Year	Country or Region	Context (ie, Site of Participants)	Types of Evidence Source (eg, Study Design)	Context of BAP Application	Discipline or Profession of BAP Use	Conceptual or Theoretic Grounding of BAP (Type)
Ghahari 2020	Canada	Community	Exploratory sequential mixed methods design	Education	Primary Care	
Gratton 2016	USA	Hospital	Unknown	Healthcare	Emergency Department Physicians	Motivational Interviewing
Gutnick 2012	International	School	Online Video	Healthcare	Mental Health	Motivational Interviewing
Gutnick et al, 2014	USA	N/A	Review of theory, literature review	Healthcare	Multidisciplinary	Motivational Interviewing
Haczkewicz 2022	Canada	Community	Randomized control trial	Health	Community Health Educators	Motivational Interviewing
Hanson et al, 2022	Canada	Clinic	Qualitative descriptive study	Healthcare	Physical Therapy	
Hesketh et al, 2021	International	Community	Parallel group randomized control group	Healthcare	Physical Therapy	
Hibbert et al, 2021	Canada	Clinic	Prospective open clinical trial, single group pre and post-test design	Healthcare	Nursing	Motivational Interviewing
Hobson & Curtis, 2017	USA	Health system	Literature Review	Healthcare	Primary Care	
Hoekstra et al, 2022	Canada	Community	Descriptive	Health	Health Coaching	Shared-Decision Making

Study	Country	Setting	Study Type	Field	Discipline	Theory/Method
Houlihan et al, 2016	USA	Community	Qualitative pilot study	Health	Health Coaching	Peer Specialists
Houlihan et al, 2017	USA	Community	Single-blinded randomized control trial	Health	Health Coaching	Peer Specialists
Huang 2020	UK	Community	In the wild study	Health	Multidisciplinary	Motivational Interviewing
Hubner & Lippke, 2014	Germany	Community	Unknown	Health	Public Health	Action Planning Theory
Ingraham et al, 2016	USA	Clinic	Pilot testing of clinician training formats	Medical Education	Quality Improvement	Motivational Interviewing
ISRCTN 2016	Canada	Clinic	Clinical trial	Health	Primary Care	Shared-Decision Making
Jacquez et al, 2018	USA	Community	Community-based participatory research	Health	Community Health Educators	Action Planning Theory
Jadotte & Lane, 2022	USA	N/A	Clinical commentary	Healthcare	Preventive Medicine	Motivational Interviewing
Jadotte-Core 2021	USA	N/A	Descriptive	Healthcare	Preventive Medicine	
Jadotte-Definitions 2021	USA	N/A	Literature Review	Healthcare	Preventive Medicine	Brief-Action Planning
Jadotte-Population, 2021	USA	School	Description of a program	Medical Education	Preventive Medicine	
Jagnnathan et al, 2018	USA	Clinic, community	Prospective cohort study	Health	Health Coaching	Motivational Interviewing
Jay et al, 2014	USA	Community	Exploratory qualitative study	Healthcare	Primary Care	Motivational Interviewing
Johnson et al, 2016	USA	Community	Non-randomized feasibility study	Healthcare	Health Coaching	

(continued on next page)

(continued)

Citation (Author-Title) Year	Country or Region	Context (ie, Site of Participants)	Types of Evidence Source (eg, Study Design)	Context of BAP Application	Discipline or Profession of BAP Use	Conceptual or Theoretic Grounding of BAP (Type)
Johnson et al, 2019	USA	Health system	Prospective cohort study	Healthcare	Community Health Educators	
Jope 2023	International	School	Workshop (Webinar)	Healthcare	Mental Health	Motivational Interviewing
Kaminetsky & Nelson 2015	USA	Clinic	Management style intervention	Healthcare	Primary Care	
Kandula et al, 2011	USA	Health system	Non-randomized pre-test, post-test study	Health	Community Health Educators	Brief Counseling
Kasidi 2022	USA	Clinic	Quality improvement	Health	Primary Care	Motivational Interviewing; Self-Efficacy
Lane & Cole 2017	USA	School	Lecture (Webinar)	Healthcare	General Medicine	Motivational Interviewing; Stages of Change
Larson & Martin 2021	USA	School	Prospective cohort study	Education	Multidisciplinary	Motivational Interviewing
Leavens et al, 2022	USA	Clinic, community	Secondary analysis of one-arm of a randomized control trial	Health	Public Health	
Leese 2009	Canada	Community	Qualitative secondary analysis of a semi-structured interview dad in mixed methods study	Healthcare	Physical Therapy	Motivational Interviewing

Leese-Ethical-Issues 2021	Canada	Community	Conceptual framework	Healthcare	Physical Therapy	
Leese-Experiences 2021	Canada	N/A	Secondary analysis of qualitative interviews nested within a randomized control trial	Healthcare	Physical Therapy	
Lewthwaite et al, 2018	USA	Clinic	Randomized control trial	Healthcare	Occupational Therapy	
Li 2018	Canada	Community	Randomized control trial	Healthcare	Physical Therapy	
Li et al, 2021	Canada	Community	Clinical Guideline Proposal	Healthcare	Physical Therapy	
Li-Community 2017	Canada	Community	Randomized control trial	Healthcare	Physical Therapy	
Li-Effects-12-wk 2020	Canada	Clinic, community	Randomized control trial with a delay-control design	Healthcare	Physical Therapy	
Li-Efficacy 2020	Canada	Health system	Randomized control trial	Healthcare	Physical Therapy	
Li-Technology 2017	Canada	Clinic	Randomized control trial	Healthcare	Physical Therapy	
Lin & Mann 2012	USA	Clinic	Intervention creation and pilot testing	Healthcare	Primary Care	Transtheoretical Model
Linzon et al, 2018	Canada	Community	Pilot study	Healthcare	Nephrology	Brief-Action Planning
Liu-Ambrose et al, 2022	Canada	Research center	Single blinded randomized control trial	Healthcare	Community Health Educators	

(continued on next page)

(continued)

Citation (Author-Title) Year	Country or Region	Context (ie, Site of Participants)	Types of Evidence Source (eg, Study Design)	Context of BAP Application	Discipline or Profession of BAP Use	Conceptual or Theoretic Grounding of BAP (Type)
Lofters et al, 2021	Canada	Community	Non-blinded randomized control trial	Healthcare	Preventive Medicine	Motivational Interviewing
Look et al, 2019	USA	Clinic	Cross-sectional stratified samples design	Healthcare	Multidisciplinary	
Lunn et al, 2019	UK	Hospital	Descriptive	Healthcare	Respiratory Clinicians	
Ly et al, 2021	Canada	Hospital, clinic	Retrospective cohort study	Healthcare	Health Coaching	Brief-Action Planning
Lynch 2016	USA	N/A	Summary Report of the Discussion from a Demonstration Video Series	Healthcare	Occupational Therapy	Motivational Interviewing
Manca et al, 2018	Canada	Clinic	Randomized control trial embedded in a mixed method design	Healthcare	Primary Care	Motivational Interviewing
Mann & Lin 2012	USA	Clinic	Clinical Trial	Healthcare	Primary Care	
Matthews et al, 2022	USA	N/A	Review of theory	Healthcare	Primary Care	
McElligot & Turnier 2020	USA	N/A	Framework overview	Education	Nursing	
Mitchell-Automated 2021	USA	Clinic	Randomized control Trial	Healthcare	Health Coaching	Motivational interviewing

Mitchell-Enabling 2021	USA	Community	Cohort study, development study	Healthcare	Health Coaching	Motivational Interviewing
Morgan-Collaborative et al, 2022	Canada	School	Curriculum map	Education	Medicine	
Morgan-Dissemination et al, 2022	Canada	Community, hospital, clinic	Systematic scoping review	Healthcare		
Murgraff et al, 2006	UK	School	Randomized control trial	Healthcare	Community Health; Addiction Medicine	
Nalder et al, 2018	Canada	Clinic, community	Exploratory qualitative study	Healthcare	Occupational Therapy	
Nault 2013	USA	Community	Randomized control trial	Healthcare	Nutrition and Exercise Science	Theory of planned behavior
NCT-Brief-Internet 2021	Canada	Community	Randomized control trial protocol	Healthcare		
NCT-Chiropractic 2015	Canada	Clinic	Clustered randomized control pilot and feasibility trial	Healthcare	Chiropractor	Self-management theory
NCT-Family-Nutrition 2014	USA	Clinic	Randomized control trial	Healthcare	Clinical Nutritionist	Motivational Interviewing
NCT-The-SOAR 2021	Canada	Community	Randomized control trial protocol	Healthcare	Physical Therapy	
Oseko 2019	Canada	Clinic			Primary Care	Motivational Interviewing

(continued on next page)

(continued)

Citation (Author-Title) Year	Country or Region	Context (ie, Site of Participants)	Types of Evidence Source (eg, Study Design)	Context of BAP Application	Discipline or Profession of BAP Use	Conceptual or Theoretic Grounding of BAP (Type)
Oshman 2017	International	School	Discussion board post	Healthcare	Primary Care	Self-Management Support
Pakpour & Sniehotta 2012	Iran	School	Prospective study	Healthcare	Public Health; Dentistry	
Park et al, 2018	Canada	Clinic, community	One group pre-post study	Healthcare	Physical Therapy	
Paszat et al, 2017	Canada	Community	Cluster randomized control trial protocol	Healthcare	Public Health	
Perkins et al, 2022	USA	Community	Cross-case analysis	Healthcare	Primary Care	
Perry et al, 2015	UK	Community, hospital, clinic	Report	Healthcare	Primary Care	
Ploughman et al, 2014	Canada	Community	Literature Review	Healthcare	Research	
Pomarensky 2022	Canada	Clinic	Literature Review	Healthcare	Physical Therapy	Motivational Interviewing
Pradhan 2014	Canada	Clinic	Scoping review, small study and survey	Healthcare	Primary Care	Self-management theory
Prior et al, 2023	Australia	Community, hospital, clinic	Systematic review with meta-analysis	Healthcare	Health Coaching	
Reims et al, 2013	USA	N/A	White paper	Healthcare, medical education		
Reims et al, 2015	USA	N/A	White paper	Healthcare, medical education		

Robin 2014	USA	Clinic	Randomized control trial	Healthcare	Primary Care; Pediatrics
Robinson et al, 2022	UK	Hospital, clinic	Machine learning assisted review of randomized control trials	Healthcare	Primary Care; Pharmacy
Rosciano & Brathwaite 2022	USA	School	Retrospective quantitative study	Healthcare	Nursing
Savarimuthu et al, 2013	USA	Health system	Plan-do-study-act	Healthcare	Multidisciplinary
Schedule 2016	USA	N/A	Workshop	Healthcare	Multidisciplinary
Schwab-Reese et al, 2021	USA	Community	Retrospective cohort study	Healthcare	Community Health; Obstetrics
Schwartz et al, 2015	USA	Health system	Cluster randomized control trial	Healthcare	Multidisciplinary
Shah et al, 2020	Canada	School	Delphi method with 2 interactions to reach consensus	Undergraduate medical education	Medical School Education
Shu et al, 2021	Canada	N/A	Single group pre-post design	Healthcare	Community Health; Peer Specialists; Physical Therapy
Siemens 2016	USA	N/A	Plan-do-study-act	Healthcare	Primary Care
Skeels et al, 2017	USA	Community	Randomized Control Trial	Health	Peer Specialists; Health Coaching
Sopcak et al, 2016	Canada	Clinic	Randomized Control Trial	Healthcare	Community Health; Peer Specialists
Sopcak et al, 2017	Canada	Clinic	Retrospective cohort study	Healthcare	Community Health; Peer Specialists
Sopcak et al, 2021	Canada	Clinic	Retrospective cohort study	Healthcare	Community Health; Peer Specialists
Sopcak et al, 2023	Canada	Clinic	Retrospective cohort study	Healthcare	Primary Care; Community Health; Nursing

(continued on next page)

(*continued*)

Citation (Author-Title) Year	Country or Region	Context (ie, Site of Participants)	Types of Evidence Source (eg, Study Design)	Context of BAP Application	Discipline or Profession of BAP Use	Conceptual or Theoretic Grounding of BAP (Type)
Stapleton 2014	Canada	Community	Randomized control trial	Health	Community Health; Peer Specialists	
Stephens 2022	Canada	Hospital	Retrospective cohort study	Healthcare	Community Health; Kinesiology	
Stephenson et al, 2018	USA	School	Retrospective cohort study	Healthcare	Clinical Nutritionist	
Tam et al, 2019	Canada	Clinic	Randomized Control Trial with delayed control design	Healthcare	Physical Therapy	
Toolkit 2015	USA	N/A	Clinical reference	Healthcare	Primary Care; Community Health	
Tumpa et al, 2019	USA	Community	Case study	Healthcare	Physical Therapy	
Tumpa 2021	USA	Health system	Pre and post cohort study	Healthcare	Physical Therapy	
Valdes et al, 2018	Canada	Clinic	Observational study	Healthcare	Physical Therapy; Occupational Therapy	
Viner et al, 2017	USA	N/A	Literature Review	Healthcare	Addiction Medicine	
Wasilewski et al, 2022	Canada	Community, hospital, clinic	Scoping Review	Health, Healthcare	Community Health	
Weisberg et al, 2021	Canada	Clinic	Case report	Healthcare	Chiropractor	
Whittaker-Feasibility-Virtual 2022	Canada	Clinic	Quasi-experimental feasibility study	Healthcare	Physical Therapy	

Whittaker-SOAR Efficacy 2022	Canada	Clinic	Two arm step wedged assessor-blinded delay-control randomized trial	Healthcare	Physical Therapy	
Whittaker-SOAR Feasibility 2022	Canada	Clinic	Quasi-experimental feasibility study	Healthcare	Physical Therapy	
Wittleder et al, 2021	USA	Clinic	Cluster-randomized trial	Healthcare	Primary Care; Health Coaching	
Wolf 2019	USA	Clinic	Randomized Control Trial	Healthcare	Clinical Nutritionist	
Yang 2021	Canada	Community	Single group pre-post design	Healthcare	Primary Care; Health Coaching	
Zerler 2017	International	Health system	Discussion board post	Healthcare	Primary Care	Motivational Interviewing

LIST OF CITATIONS OF INCLUDED STUDIES

Allin S, Shepherd J, Munce S, et al. Online health coaching for Canadians with spinal cord injury: SCI&U pilot Results [Journal article; Conference proceeding]. Journal of spinal cord medicine 2019;42:S252.

Allin S, Shepherd J, Thorson T, et al. Web-Based Health Coaching for Spinal Cord Injury: Results From a Mixed Methods Feasibility Evaluation. JMIR Rehabilitation and Assistive Technologies 2020;7(2). https://doi.org/10.2196/16351.

American Psychiatric Association. Hybrid online introductory brief action plan 2022. Retrieved March 15 from. https://motivationalinterviewing.org/hybrid-online-introductory-brief-action-plan.

Applegate M, Scott E, Taksler GB, et al. Project ACTIVE: a randomized controlled trial of personalized and patient-centered preventive care in an urban safety-net setting. J Gen Intern Med 2021;36:606–13.

Ayyoub L, Hvizd A, Grace S, et al. Glucofit: A pilot study evaluating a brief action planning intervention in individuals with type 2 diabetes following a community-based physical activity program. Journal of Exercise, Movement, and Sport (SCAPPS refereed abstracts repository) 2017;49(1):148.

Brathwaite B, Marino M, Bruckenthal P. Nurse Practitioner Confidence and Attitudes towards Brief Motivational Interventions to Improve Compliance with Health and Wellness Recommendations. J Comm Pub Health Nursing 2018;4(212):2.

Brody M, Houlihan BV, Skeels SE, et al. Development of a peer-led phone intervention for goal-setting health care needs in spinal cord injury [Journal article; Conference proceeding]. ARCHIVES OF PHYSICAL MEDICINE AND REHABILITATION 2015; 96(10):e19. https://www.cochranelibrary.com/central/doi/10.1002/central/CN-01126827/full.

Bruckenthal P. 1F A Taste of MI: Motivational Interviewing and Brief Action Planning for Pain Management Nurses.28th National Conference of American Society for Pain Management Nursing, September 26-29 2018, Bonita Springs, Florida. Pain Manag Nurs 2019;20(2):95.

Clayton C, Feehan L, Goldsmith CH, et al. Feasibility and preliminary efficacy of a physical activity counseling intervention using Fitbit in people with knee osteoarthritis: the TRACK-OA study protocol. Pilot and Feasibility Studies 2015;1.

Cole S. Brief action planning (Video): a practical MI tool for primary care 2012. Retrieved March 15 from. https://motivationalinterviewing.org/forum/brief-action-planning-video-practical-mi-tool-primary-care.

Cole S. MI MED living registry 2021. Retrieved March 15 from. https://live-mint-d7-upgraded.pantheonsite.io/sites/default/files/05.07.21_mi_med_-_living_registry_responses_-_form_responses_1.pdf.

Cole S, Bogenschutz M, Hungerford D. Motivational interviewing and psychiatry: Use in addiction treatment, risky drinking and routine practice. Focus 2011;9(1):42–54.

Cole, S., Cole, M. D., Gutnick, D., et al (2013). Function three: collaborate for management. The medical interview E-book: the three function approach, 34.

Cole, S., Gutnick, D., & Weiner, J. (2013). Stepped-care advanced skills for action planning. The medical interview E-book: the three function approach, 125.

Connell G, Verville L, Cancelliere C, et al. Brief action planning targeting prognostic factors for an adult with persistent low back pain without radiculopathy: A case report. Clinical Case Reports 2020;8(12):2776–80.

Davis, C. (2012). An introduction to quality improvement for MINTies. Retrieved March 15 from https://live-mint-d7-upgraded.pantheonsite.io/sites/default/files/2012QI 4MINT.pdf.

Davis, C. (2017). How Long Does It Take to Use Patient-Centered Communication? Institute for Healthcare Improvement. Retrieved March 15 from https://www.ihi. org/education/IHIOpenSchool/resources/Pages/A udioandVideo/ConnieDavis-HowLongDoesItTakeToUsePatientCenteredCommunication.aspx.

Deegala C, Champany R. 2017 continuing dental education catalog - general courses - DE0028: motivational interviewing. Indian health Service 2017. Retrieved March 15 from. https://www.ihs.gov/dentalcde/index.cfm?fuseaction=catalog.printcat alog&year=2017.

Dhopte P, French SD, Quon JA, et al. Guideline implementation in the Canadian chiropractic setting: a pilot cluster randomized controlled trial and parallel study. Chiropr Man Ther 2019;27. https://doi.org/10.1186/s12998-019-0253-z. Article 31.

Duncan-Carnesciali J, Wallace BC, Odlum M. An evaluation of a diabetes self-management education (DSME) intervention delivered using avatar-based technology: Certified diabetes educators' ratings and perceptions. Diabetes Educat 2018; 44(3):216–24.

Eilayyan O. Optimizing Primary Healthcare Professional Practices in Chronic Low Back Pain Management (Publication Number 28250518) [Ph.D., McGill University (Canada)]. Canada – Quebec, CA: ProQuest dissertations & theses global; 2017.

Eilayyan O, Thomas A, Hallé MC, et al. Promoting the use of self-management in novice chiropractors treating individuals with spine pain: the design of a theory-based knowledge translation intervention. BMC Musculoskelet Disord 2018; 19(1):328.

Eilayyan O, Thomas A, Hallé MC, et al. Promoting the use of self-management in patients with spine pain managed by chiropractors and chiropractic interns: barriers and design of a theory-based knowledge translation intervention. Chiropr Man Therap 2019;27:44.

Falck RS, Best JR, Li LC, et al. Can we improve cognitive function among adults with osteoarthritis by increasing moderate-to-vigorous physical activity and reducing sedentary behaviour? Secondary analysis of the MONITOR-OA study. BMC Muscoskel Disord 2018;19. https://doi.org/10.1186/s12891-018-2369-z.

Falck RS, Davis JC, Best JR, et al. Effect of a multimodal lifestyle intervention on sleep and cognitive function in older adults with probable mild cognitive impairment and poor sleep: a randomized clinical trial. J Alzheim Dis 2020;76(1):179–93.

Falck RS, Davis JC, Best JR, et al. Buying time: a proof-of-concept randomized controlled trial to improve sleep quality and cognitive function among older adults with mild cognitive impairment. Trials 2018;19(1):1–9.

Farmer AJ, Oke J, Hardeman W, et al. The effect of a brief action planning intervention on adherence to double-blind study medication, compared to a standard trial protocol, in the Atorvastatin in Factorial with Omega EE90 Risk Reduction in Diabetes (AFORRD) clinical trial: A cluster randomised sub-study. Diabetes Res Clin Pract 2016;120:56–64.

Gainforth HL. The Role of Communication Channels for Knowledge Mobilization in a Community-Based Organization (Publication Number 28389615) [Ph.D., Queen's University (Canada)]. Canada – Ontario, CA: ProQuest dissertations & theses global; 2013.

Galaviz KI, Narayan KV, Lobelo F, et al. Lifestyle and the prevention of type 2 diabetes: a status report. Am J Lifestyle Med 2018;12(1):4–20.

Gallegos-Carrillo K, García-Peña C, Salmerón J, et al. Brief counseling and exercise referral scheme: a pragmatic trial in Mexico. Am J Prev Med 2017;52(2):249–59.

Gaughan M, Brinckman D. Telephonic Health Coaching (THC) Promotes Health Behavior Changes Among Participants in SNAP-Ed. J Nutr Educ Behav 2017;49(7, Supplement 1):S98.

Gaughan M, Brinckman D. P86 - SNAP-Ed: A Platform for Teaching Motivational Interviewing and Behavior Change Skills. J Nutr Educ Behav 2018;50(7, Supplement):S71.

Ghahari, S, Burnett, S, & Alexander, L. (2020). Development and pilot testing of a health education program to improve immigrants' access to Canadian health services. BMC Health Services Research, 20, 1-12. https://doi.org/10.1186/s12913-020-05180-y.

Gratton, P. (2016). A Phenomenological Investigation of Factors Leading to Success in Diverting Non-Urgent Emergency Department Use at a Rural Critical Access Hospital Using the Patient Centered Medical Home Model. https://digitalcommons.georgefox.edu/dbadmin/9.

Gutnick, D. (2012). Engaging Primary Care Providers in discussions about MI - Mr. Smith's Smoking Evolution You tube video. Retrieved March 15 from https://motivationalinterviewing.org/forum/engaging-primary-care-providers-discussions-about-mi-mr-smiths-smoking-evolution-you-tube-vide.

Gutnick D, Reims K, Davis C, et al. Brief Action Planning to Facilitate Behavior Change and Support Patient Self-Management. J Clin Outcome Manag 2014;21(1):17–29. http://proxy.library.stonybrook.edu/login?url=https://search.ebscohost.com/login.aspx?direct=true&db=rzh&AN=93882314&site=ehost-live&scope=site.

Haczkewicz KM. *The effectiveness of a brief internet-delivered behaviour change intervention among health middle-aged adults: a randomized controlled trial* Faculty of Arts. University of Regina; 2022.

Hanson HM, Friesen J, Beaupre L, et al. Supporting Rehabilitation of Rural Patients Receiving Total Knee Arthroplasty Through Physical Activity: Perceptions of Stakeholder Groups. ACR Open Rheumatology 2022;4(10):863–71.

Hesketh K, Low J, Andrews R, et al. Mobile Health Biometrics to Enhance Exercise and Physical Activity Adherence in Type 2 Diabetes (MOTIVATE-T2D): protocol for a feasibility randomised controlled trial. BMJ Open 2021;11(11):e052563.

Hibbert C, Trottier E, Boville M, et al. The effect of peer support on knowledge and self-efficacy in weight management: a prospective clinical trial in a mental health setting. Community Ment Health J 2021;57:979–84.

Hobson A, Curtis A. Improving the care of veterans: The role of nurse practitioners in team-based population health management. Journal of the American association of Nurse Practitioners 2017;29(11):644–50.

Hoekstra F, Collins D, Dinwoodie M, et al. Measuring behavior change technique delivery and receipt in physical activity behavioral interventions. Rehabil Psychol 2022;67(2):128.

Houlihan BV, Brody M, Everhart-Skeels S, et al. Randomized Trial of a Peer-Led, Telephone-Based Empowerment Intervention for Persons With Chronic Spinal Cord Injury Improves Health Self-Management. Archives of physical medicine and rehabilitation 2017;98(6):1067–76.e1061.

Houlihan BV, Everhart-Skeels S, Gutnick D, et al. Empowering Adults With Chronic Spinal Cord Injury to Prevent Secondary Conditions. Arch PM&R (Phys Med Rehabil) 2016;97(10):1687–95.e1685.

Huang Y. Internet of Things enabled sedentary behaviour change in office workers: development and feasibility of a novel intervention. *WorkMyWay)* University of Nottingham; 2020.

Hübner G, Lippke S. Investigating and promoting the decision towards signing an organ donation card. Open J Med Psychol 2014.

Ingraham N, Magrini D, Brooks J, et al. Two Tailored Provider Curricula Promoting Healthy Weight in Lesbian and Bisexual Women. Wom Health Issues 2016;26: S36–42.

Isrctn. (2016). BETTER prevention and screening: personalized clinical visits for adults Trial registry record; Clinical trial protocol. https://trialsearch.who.int/Trial2.aspx?TrialID=ISRCTN21333761. https://www.cochranelibrary.com/central/doi/10.1002/central/CN-01817909/full.

Jacquez F, Vaughn LM, Suarez-Cano G. Implementation of a Stress Intervention with Latino Immigrants in a Non-traditional Migration City. J Immigr Minority Health 2019; 21(2):372–82.

Jadotte YT, Lane DS. Core functions, knowledge bases and essential services: A proposed prescription for the evolution of the preventive medicine specialty. Prev Med 2021;143:106286.

Jadotte YT, Lane DS. Population health rounds: A novel vehicle for training in population medicine and clinical preventive medicine. J Publ Health Manag Pract 2021;27(1):S139–45.

Jadotte YT, Muzaffar S, Zaza S. Preparedness in Routine Prevention: Levers for the Preventive Medicine Specialty in the Healthcare Context. Am J Prev Med 2022; 62(4):656–60.

Jadotte YT, Noel K. Definitions and core competencies for interprofessional education in telehealth practice. Clinics in Integrated Care 2021;6:100054.

Jagannathan R, Ziolkowski SL, Weber MB, et al. Physical activity promotion for patients transitioning to dialysis using the "Exercise is Medicine" framework: a multi centor randomized pragmatic trial (EIM-CKD trial) protocol. BMC Nephrol 2018; 19. https://doi.org/10.1186/s12882-018-1032 0.

Jay M, Gutnick D, Squires A, et al. In our country tortilla doesn't make us fat: cultural factors influencing lifestyle goal-setting for overweight and obese urban, Latina patients. J Health Care Poor Underserved 2014;25(4):1603.

Johnson HM, LaMantia JN, Warner RC, et al. MyHEART: a non randomized feasibility study of a young adult hypertension intervention. Journal of hypertension and management 2016;2(2).

Johnson HM, Sullivan-Vedder L, Kim K, et al. Rationale and study design of the MyHEART study: A young adult hypertension self-management randomized controlled trial. Contemp Clin Trials 2019;78:88–100.

Jope, B. (2023). Advanced motivational interviewing. Retrieved March 15 from https://motivationalinterviewing.org/facilitator-led-online-advanced-77.

Kaminetzky CP, Nelson KM. In the office and in-between: the role of panel management in primary care. J Gen Intern Med 2015;30:876–7.

Kandula NR, Malli T, Zei CP, et al. Literacy and retention of information after a multimedia diabetes education program and teach-back. J Health Commun 2011; 16(sup3):89–102.

Kasidi J. Quality Improvement Project Utilizing a Comprehensive Toolkit with Individualized Food Label Education and Brief Action Planning for Healthy Food Choices to Reduce the Burden of Chronic Disease Among Black People in the United States. Nursing research 2022;71(3):S104.

Lane, S., & Cole, S. (2017). Motivational interviewing and brief action planning for smoking cessation in primary care. NY Chapter of the American College of Physicians. Retrieved March 15 from https://www.nyacp.org/i4a/pages/index.cfm?pageid=3794.

Larson E, Martin BA. Measuring motivational interviewing self-efficacy of pre-service students completing a competency-based motivational interviewing course. Exploratory Research in Clinical and Social Pharmacy 2021;1:100009.

Leavens EL, Nollen NL, Ahluwalia JS, et al. Changes in dependence, withdrawal, and craving among adult smokers who switch to nicotine salt pod-based e-cigarettes. Addiction 2022;117(1):207–15.

Leese J. Self-managing with physical activity wearables: emerging ethical issues from the perspectives of persons living with *arthritis*. University of British Columbia; 2021.

Leese J, MacDonald G, Backman CL, et al. Experiences of Wearable Technology by Persons with Knee Osteoarthritis Participating in a Physical Activity Counseling Intervention: Qualitative Study Using a Relational Ethics Lens. JMIR mHealth and uHealth 2021;9(11). https://doi.org/10.2196/30332.

Leese J, Zhu S, Townsend AF, et al. Ethical issues experienced by persons with rheumatoid arthritis in a wearable-enabled physical activity intervention study. Health Expect 2022;25(4):1418–31.

Lewthwaite R, Winstein CJ, Lane CJ, et al. Accelerating stroke recovery: body structures and functions, activities, participation, and quality of life outcomes from a large rehabilitation trial. Neurorehabilitation Neural Repair 2018;32(2):150–65.

Li LC, Feehan LM, Hoens AM. Rethinking physical activity promotion during the COVID-19 pandemic: Focus on a 24-hour day. J Rheumatol 2021;48:1205–7.

Li LC, Feehan LM, Shaw C, et al. A technology-enabled Counselling program versus a delayed treatment control to support physical activity participation in people with inflammatory arthritis: study protocol for the OPAM-IA randomized controlled trial. BMC Rheumatology 2017;1:1–8.

Li LC, Feehan LM, Xie H, et al. Efficacy of a physical activity counseling program with use of a wearable tracker in people with inflammatory arthritis: a randomized controlled trial. Arthritis Care Res 2020;72(12):1755–65.

Li LC, Feehan LM, Xie H, et al. Effects of a 12-Week Multifaceted Wearable-Based Program for People With Knee Osteoarthritis: Randomized Controlled Trial. JMIR mHealth and uHealth 2020;8(7). https://doi.org/10.2196/19116.

Li LC, Sayre EC, Xie H, et al. A Community-Based Physical Activity Counselling Program for People With Knee Osteoarthritis: Feasibility and Preliminary Efficacy of the Track-OA Study. JMIR Health and Health 2017;5(6). https://doi.org/10.2196/mhealth.7863.

Li LC, Sayre EC, Xie H, et al. Efficacy of a community-based technology-enabled physical activity counseling program for people with knee osteoarthritis: proof-of-concept study. J Med Internet Res 2018;20(4):e159.

Lin JJ, Mann DM. Application of persuasion and health behavior theories for behavior change counseling: Design of the ADAPT (Avoiding Diabetes Thru Action Plan Targeting) program. Patient Educ Counsel 2012;88(3):460–6.

Linzon R, Gray BG, Chan A, et al. Brief Action Planning (BAP): A Self-Management Support Technique for Promoting Collaborative Goal Setting for Patients on Home Dialysis. Am J Kidney Dis 2017;69(4):A64.

Liu-Ambrose T, Falck RS, Dao E, et al. Effect of Exercise Training or Complex Mental and Social Activities on Cognitive Function in Adults With Chronic Stroke: A Randomized Clinical Trial. JAMA Netw Open 2022;5(10):e2236510.

Lofters AK, O'Brien MA, Sutradhar R, et al. Building on existing tools to improve chronic disease prevention and screening in public health: a cluster randomized trial. BMC Publ Health 2021;21:1–11.

Look M, Kolotkin RL, Dhurandhar NV, et al. Implications of differing attitudes and experiences between providers and persons with obesity: results of the national ACTION study. PGM (Postgrad Med) 2019;131(5):357–65.

Lunn S, Dharmagunawardena R, Lander M, et al. It's hard to talk about breathlessness: a unique insight from respiratory trainees. Clin Med 2019;19(4):344.

Ly M, Stephens S, Iruthayanathan R, et al. Physical Activity in Youth with Multiple Sclerosis receiving the ATOMIC intervention: Social connectedness above all else. Multiple Sclerosis and Related Disorders 2021;49:102795.

Lynch, H. (2016). Discussion Options for Change Planning. Retrieved March 15 from https://motivationalinterviewing.org/forum/mi-emerging-era-telemedicine-request-references-slide-sets-ideas.

Manca DP, Fernandes C, Grunfeld E, et al. The BETTER WISE protocol: building on existing tools to improve cancer and chronic disease prevention and screening in primary care for wellness of cancer survivors and patients – a cluster randomized controlled trial embedded in a mixed methods design. BMC Cancer 2018;18. https://doi.org/10.1186/s12885-018-4839-y.

Mann DM, Lin JJ. Increasing efficacy of primary care-based counseling for diabetes prevention: Rationale and design of the ADAPT (Avoiding Diabetes Thru Action Plan Targeting) trial. Implement Sci 2012;7:6.

Matthews JA, DBH M, NBC-HWC D, et al. A Coach Approach to Facilitating Behavior Change. J Fam Pract 2022;71(1 Suppl Lifestyle):eS93–9.

McElligott D, Turnier J. Integrative Health and Wellness Assessment Tool. Crit Care Nurs Clin 2020;32(3):439–50.

Mitchell EG. Enabling automated, conversational health coaching with human-centered artificial intelligence (publication number 28721586) [ph.D., Columbia university. United States – New York: ProQuest Dissertations & Theses Global; 2021.

Mitchell EG, Maimone R, Cassells A, et al. Automated vs. human health coaching: Exploring participant and practitioner experiences. Proceedings of the ACM on human-computer interaction 2021;5(CSCW1):1–37.

Mitchell, E. G., Maimone, R., & Mamykina, L. (2020). Characterizing Human vs. Automated Coaching: Preliminary Results. Extended Abstracts of the 2020 CHI Conference on Human Factors in Computing Systems.

Morgan TL, Nowlan Suart T, Fortier MS, et al. Moving toward co-production: five ways to get a grip on collaborative implementation of Movement Behaviour curricula in undergraduate medical education. Canadian Medical Education Journal 2022; 13(5):87–100.

Morgan TL, Romani C, Ross-White A, et al. Dissemination and implementation strategies for physical activity guidelines among adults with disability, chronic conditions, and pregnancy: a systematic scoping review. BMC Publ Health 2022;22:1–38.

Murgraff V, McDermott D, Abraham C. An evaluation of an action-planning intervention to reduce the incidence of high-risk single-session alcohol consumption in high risk drinkers. End of Award Report to the Alcohol Education and Research Council on Grant(71D); 2006. p. M212.

Nalder E, Marziali E, Dawson DR, et al. Delivering cognitive behavioural interventions in an internet-based healthcare delivery environment. Br J Occup Ther 2018; 81(10):591–600.

Nault, E. M. (2013). Theory of Planned Behavior: Item Response Sets and Prediction of Physical Activity Virginia Tech.

Nct. (2014). Family Nutrition Physical Activity Tool Use During Well Child Visits Trial registry record; Clinical trial protocol. https://clinicaltrials.gov/show/NCT02067728. https://www.cochranelibrary.com/central/doi/10.1002/central/CN-01543824/full.

Nct. (2015). Testing the Feasibility of Intervening to Optimize Chiropractic Care for Adults With Neck Pain Disorders Trial registry record; Clinical trial protocol. https://clinicaltrials.gov/show/NCT02483091. https://www.cochranelibrary.com/central/doi/10.1002/central/CN-02033010/full.

Nct. (2021). Effectiveness of a Brief Internet-delivered Behaviour Change Intervention Among Healthy Middle-aged Adults Trial registry record; Clinical trial protocol. https://clinicaltrials.gov/show/NCT05033184. https://www.cochranelibrary.com/central/doi/10.1002/central/CN-02307678/full.

Nct. (2021). The SOAR (Stop OsteoARthritis) Program Proof-of-Concept Study Trial registry record; Clinical trial protocol. https://clinicaltrials.gov/show/NCT04956393. https://www.cochranelibrary.com/central/doi/10.1002/central/CN-02290258/full.

Oseko E. Primary care SERVICE IN adult mental health 2019.

Oshman, L. (2017). Brief action planning and autonomy. Retrieved March 15 from https://motivationalinterviewing.org/forum/brief-action-planning-and-autonomy.

Pakpour AH, Sniehotta FF. Perceived behavioural control and coping planning predict dental brushing behaviour among Iranian adolescents. J Clin Periodontol 2012; 39(2):132–7.

Park C, Sayre EC, Li LC. Feasibility and Preliminary-efficacy of a Multi-faceted Physical Activity Counselling Program for Persons with Knee Osteoarthritis. J Rheumatol 2018.

Paszat L, Sutradhar R, Mary Ann OB, et al. BETTER HEALTH: Durham – protocol for a cluster randomized trial of BETTER in community and public health settings. BMC Publ Health 2017;17:1.

Perkins A, Bradley A, Magaldi J. Case analyses of state-sponsored asthma quality improvement interventions–benefits and technical assistance efforts. J Asthma 2022;59(3):616–27.

Perry C, Chhatralia K, Damesick D, et al. Behavioural insights in health care. London: The Health Foundation; 2015. p. 18–29.

Ploughman M, Deshpande N, Latimer-Cheung AE, et al. Drawing on related knowledge to advance multiple sclerosis falls-prevention research. International journal of MS care 2014;16(4):163–70.

Pomarensky M. Athletic therapist's management of persistent musculoskeletal pain: Time to embrace a biopsychosocial lens. J Athl Train 2021.

Pradhan P. Evaluating Readiness to Change Health Behaviours in Individuals with Chronic Pain (Publication Number 28265646) [M.Sc., McGill University (Canada)]. Canada – Quebec, CA: ProQuest dissertations & theses global; 2014.

Prior JL, Vesentini G, Michell De Gregorio JA, et al. Health Coaching for Low Back Pain and Hip and Knee Osteoarthritis: A Systematic Review with Meta-Analysis. Pain Med 2023;24(1):32–51.

Reims, K., Gutnick, D., Davis, C., et al (2015). Brief action planning white paper. 2012. In.

Reims K, Gutnick D, Davis C, et al. Brief action planning. Centre for collaboration, motivation and innovation; 2013.

Robin R. Brief Action Planning Paired with Obesigenic Screening in Pediatric Primary Care Clinics: Description of Methods and Design. 2014. AAP national conference and exhibition; 2014.

Robinson L, Arden M, Dawson S, et al. A machine-learning assisted review of the use of habit formation in medication adherence interventions for long-term conditions. Health Psychol Rev 2022;1–23.

Rosciano A, Brathwaite B. Sexual Well-Being and Screening for Risky Sexual Behaviors: A Quantitative Retrospective Study. Journal of the New York State Nurses Association 2022;49(1):28–37.

Savarimuthu SM, Jensen AE, Schoenthaler A, et al. Developing a toolkit for panel management: improving hypertension and smoking cessation outcomes in primary care at the VA. BMC Fam Pract 2013;14:176.

Schedule, D. (2016). Intermediate to advanced motivational interviewing for skill development & Supervision.

Schwab-Reese LM, Renner LM, King H, et al. "They're very passionate about making sure that women stay healthy": a qualitative examination of women's experiences participating in a community paramedicine program. BMC Health Serv Res 2021; 21:1–13.

Schwartz MD, Jensen A, Wang B, et al. Panel management to improve smoking and hypertension outcomes by VA primary care teams: a cluster-randomized controlled trial. J Gen Intern Med 2015;30:916–23.

Shah S, McCann M, Yu C. Developing a National Competency-Based Diabetes Curriculum in Undergraduate Medical Education: A Delphi Study. Can J Diabetes 2020;44(1):30–6.e32.

Shu H, Ginis KM, Levett CLC, et al. Physical activity coaching implementation among physiotherapists and SCI peer mentors: behavioural determinants and effects 2021.

Siemens AC. Improving Patient Care Delivery in a Small Alaska Native Health Care Organization (Publication Number 3746361) [Ph.D., Walden University]. United States – Minnesota: Ethnic NewsWatch; ProQuest dissertations & theses global; 2016.

Skeels S, Pernigotti D, Houlihan B, et al. SCI peer health coach influence on self-management with peers: a qualitative analysis. Spinal Cord 2017;55(11):1016–22.

Sopcak N, Aguilar C, Nykiforuk CI, et al. Patients' perspectives on BETTER 2 prevention and screening: qualitative findings from Newfoundland & Labrador. BJGP open 2017;1(3).

Sopcak N, Aguilar C, Obrien MA, et al. Implementation of the BETTER 2 program: a qualitative study exploring barriers and facilitators of a novel way to improve chronic disease prevention and screening in primary care. Implement Sci 2016; 11. https://doi.org/10.1186/s13012-016-0525-0.

Sopcak N, Fernandes C, O'Brien MA, et al. What is a prevention visit? A qualitative study of a structured approach to prevention and screening – the BETTER WISE project. BMC Fam Pract 2021;22:1–11.

Sopcak N, Wong M, Fernandes C, et al. Prevention and screening during the COVID-19 pandemic: qualitative findings from the BETTER WISE project. BMC Primary Care 2023;24(1):27.

Stapleton, J. (2014). A systematic examination of the role of social influence on leisure time physical activity among persons with physical disabilities.

Stephens S, Schneiderman JE, Finlayson M, et al. Feasibility of a theory-informed mobile app for changing physical activity in youth with multiple sclerosis. Multiple Sclerosis and Related Disorders 2022;58:103467.

Stephenson T, Gustafson A, Houlihan J, et al. The obesity food insecurity paradox: Student focus group feedback to guide development of innovative curriculum. J Nutr Educ Behav 2018;50(7):S71–2.

Tam J, Lacaille D, Liu-Ambrose T, et al. Effectiveness of an online self-management tool, OPERAS (an On-demand Program to EmpoweR Active Self-management), for people with rheumatoid arthritis: a research protocol. Durham: Research Square; 2019.

Toolkit, U. P. AHRQ Health Literacy Universal Precautions Toolkit.

Tumpa J, Ahamed S, Cole S, et al. The Development of Electronic Brief Action Planning (E-BAP): A Self-Management Support Tool for Health Behavior Change. 41st annual meeting of the society for medical decision making; 2019.

Tumpa JF. Explainable retinal screening with self-management support to improve eye-health of diabetic population via telemedicine (publication number 28866428) [ph.D., marquette university]. United States – Wisconsin: ProQuest Dissertations & Theses Global; 2021.

Valdés BA, Glegg SM, Lambert-Shirzad N, et al. Application of commercial games for home-based rehabilitation for people with hemiparesis: challenges and lessons learned. Game Health J 2018;7(3):197–207.

Viner J, Viner L, Monroe-Cook D. Minding the Brain: A developmental neurobiological model for substance abuse treatment in emerging adults. Yellow Brick J Emerg Adulthood 2017;3:13–8.

Wasilewski MB, Rios J, Simpson R, et al. Peer support for traumatic injury survivors: a scoping review. Disabil Rehabil 2022;1–34.

Weisberg J, Connell G, Verville L, et al. Brief action planning to facilitate the management of acute low back pain with radiculopathy and yellow flags: a case report. J Can Chiropr Assoc 2021;65(2):212–8.

Whittaker JL, Truong LK, Losciale JM, et al. Efficacy of the SOAR knee health program: protocol for a two-arm stepped-wedge randomized delayed-controlled trial. BMC Muscoskel Disord 2022;23:1–13.

Whittaker JL, Truong LK, Losciale JM, et al. Feasibility of a virtual, physiotherapist-guided knee health program to manage osteoarthritis risk after an activity-related knee injury. Osteoarthritis Cartilage 2022;30:S224–5.

Whittaker JL, Truong LK, Silvester-Lee T, et al. Feasibility of the SOAR (Stop OsteoARthritis) program. Osteoarthritis and Cartilage Open 2022;4(1):100239.

Wittleder S, Smith S, Wang B, et al. Peer-Assisted Lifestyle (PAL) intervention: a protocol of a cluster-randomised controlled trial of a health-coaching intervention delivered by veteran peers to improve obesity treatment in primary care. BMJ Open 2021;11(2). https://doi.org/10.1136/bmjopen-2020-043013.

Wolf T. Chronic Disease Prevention: Nutrition and Behavioral Neuroscience Approaches (Publication Number 22587390) [Ph.D., Iowa State University]. United States – Iowa: ProQuest dissertations & theses global; 2019.

Yang MC. Understanding chronic disease management in older adults during the COVID-19. *pandemic* University of British Columbia; 2021.

Zerler, H. (2017). Observation Coaching and Feedback in Primary Care settings. Retrieved March 15 from https://motivationalinterviewing.org/forum/observation-coaching-and-feedback-primary-care-settings.

Mobile Health and Preventive Medicine

Jill Waalen, MD, MS, MPH

KEYWORDS

- Mobile health • Preventive medicine • Prevention • Digital medicine • Sensors
- Activity trackers • Electrocardiogram monitors • Continuous glucose monitoring

KEY POINTS

- The development of wearable devices that provide health-related data (mobile health or mHealth) relevant to prevention has a long history, starting with pedometers, with roots in centuries past.
- Technological advances, accelerated by smartphones and smartwatches, have brought a wide array of mHealth, modalities to the fingertips of millions, with many more devices providing data of all types to come.
- Research on the application of mHealth to preventive medicine is most mature for devices including activity trackers, electrocardiogram monitors, and continuous glucose monitors that are highlighted in this article.
- Lessons learned include the need for continued integration of mHealth technologies, including those related to behavior change, to maximize its impact on prevention, as the concepts of digital health coaching and hospital-at-home advance.

Since the introduction of wearable devices that generate personal health data, the potential for their use in prevention has been met with great enthusiasm. From the introduction of wrist-worn devices ushered in by the Fitbit craze of the 2010s–along with the 10,000 steps mantra—to the more recent advent of the mobile electrocardiogram (ECG), continuous glucose monitors, and an ever-growing list of other devices, preventive medicine-related applications have expanded beyond personal fitness to early detection and disease management. At the same time, technology has continued to advance, creating devices that are increasingly smaller, less obtrusive and more accurate. Although the term "mobile" in mobile health (mHealth) once referred to devices that could theoretically be used at home—such as Holter monitors and ambulatory blood pressure cuffs–mHealth now affords convenient and continuous monitoring of various physiologic processes passively, requiring little effort or inconvenience to the user.

University of California, San Diego/San Diego State University General Preventive Medicine Residency Program & Scripps Research Translational Institute, 3344 North Torrey Pines Court, La Jolla, CA 92037, USA
E-mail address: jwaalen@scripps.edu

Med Clin N Am 107 (2023) 1097–1108
https://doi.org/10.1016/j.mcna.2023.06.003
0025-7125/23/© 2023 Elsevier Inc. All rights reserved.

medical.theclinics.com

For all the advancements and proliferation of personal wearable devices delivering health-related data, challenges remain for mHealth to have a large-scale impact on personal and population health. The availability of data flowing from these devices does not always translate into their use for guiding healthful behavior. There is also a significant lag between the often splashy market introduction of these devices and the development of a sufficient evidence base on their effectiveness and best strategies for their use in impacting health outcomes. Use of these data by health care providers has also lagged, with the literature mostly limited to feasibility studies to date.

In this review, three of the currently most widely used and studied mHealth technologies are highlighted in the major domains of preventive medicine as examples of the realized potential, the common challenges in their effective application in prevention, and the new measures of health and disease they are introducing. The many smart sensors along with the accompanying artificial intelligence (AI) that are in various stages of development are also previewed with their potential to further transform mHealth and preventive medicine to improve human health.

PRIMARY PREVENTION: ACTIVITY TRACKERS TO INCREASE PHYSICAL FITNESS FOR PEOPLE OF ALL AGES AND HEALTH STATUS
A Brief History

The personal activity tracker has one of the longest histories as a prototypic mHealth device, beginning with the pedometer, a purely mechanical device for counting steps. One of the earliest of these, designed by Leonardo da Vinci, involved a lever attached to the thigh, with later versions using a string attached to the knee. By the 1820s, Swiss watchmakers had developed mechanisms that could be included in watch-sized devices using spring-suspended lever arms to detect motion.[1] As refinements continued, the daily goal of 10,000 steps originated with the Japanese pedometer maker Yamasa in 1965; an electronic pedometer with a digital display came from the same company 1990. With the introduction of the first wrist-worn devices by companies such as Fitbit, Jawbone, and Garmin, among many others in 2009, the popularity of activity tracking (along with the 10,000 step mantra), skyrocketed and soon the technology was available in smartphones and smartwatches.

As one of the oldest examples of mHealth, these devices also have the longest track record of study, with the expected health benefits based on the simple premise that activity measured by the device translates into energy expenditure, the tracking of which can promote increased activity, leading to fitness and weight loss. Given the numerous studies that have been performed on each aspect of that premise, a clear picture of the effects of these devices is available.

Device Accuracy and Impact in Randomized Controlled Trials

Numerous studies have shown the accuracy of these devices is highest for step counts, with much more variability within and between devices in measures of distance, physical activity level, and energy expenditure.[2–5] Despite the imprecision of its translation into energy expenditure, the measure of steps, which represent a major form of daily physical activity, has been considered useful in promoting that activity. Some of the cited advantages of the step count as such a measure of physical activity are that they

Are objective, intuitive, and easy to understand for laypeople and translatable into motivational and public health messages
Are useful for categorizing people into less active and more active categories

Have strong associations with physical health variables[1]

In fact, multiple randomized controlled trials (RCTs) have found that they influence activity levels and some physiological measures in a positive direction in various populations of all ages and levels of health. A recent comprehensive umbrella review encompassing systematic reviews and meta-analyses representing a total of 390 RCTs including nearly 164,000 participants across all age groups summarized various outcomes.[6] These studies showed that use of wearable activity trackers significantly increased physical activity, with effect sizes ranging from 0.3 to 0.6, translating into an increase of 1800 steps per day, 40 minutes per day of walking time, and 6 minutes per day of moderate-to-vigorous physical activity. Increases in physical activity were found to occur in all age groups, from children to older adults, and among groups with different levels of baseline health, including healthy participants, as well as those with diabetes, cardiovascular disease, obesity, Alzheimer disease and other conditions.

Activity trackers have also been shown to have positive, although generally smaller, effects in studies with physiological outcomes. The strongest evidence was seen for weight loss, of 0.5 to 1.5 kg over time of use, decrease in waist circumference of around 1.5 cm, decreased body mass index (BMI) of 0.5 kg/m^2, and increased aerobic capacity measured by maximum oxygen consumption (VO$_2$ max) of 1.7 mL/kg/min.[6] Decreases in systolic blood pressure and heart rate were also found by most studies included in the meta-analyses, but with less consistency and a lesser effect. Studies on effects of activity tracker use on diastolic blood pressure, cholesterol, triglycerides, hemoglobin A1C (A1C), and fasting glucose reported effects that were not statistically significant. Studies on the duration of effects on increasing physical activity showed strong effects maintained over 4 to 6 months, with diminished but still significant effects as far out as 4 years in 1 study. Effects on body composition were less robust or long lasting. Results of studies regarding psychosocial effects and quality of life have been mostly inconclusive.[6–10]

Toward Increasing Real-World Impact

The overall conclusions from RCTs involving usage of activity trackers from several months to several years, are that they are an effective intervention to increase physical activity, regardless of how accurate the measures, with resultant positive effects of weight loss, decreased BMI, and increased VO$_2$ max, with less effect on other physiologic parameters. Study participants with illnesses appeared to be more motivated by activity tracker interventions overall.[6]

The decrease in effect in promoting activity and in use of the devices in general over time by individuals observed even in the relatively controlled setting of these clinical trials, however, begs the question of what effect these devices have in the real-world setting. Although uptake of commercial products has been robust, abandonment of these devices is common, limiting their potential for lasting effects on personal health and on a population level as evidenced by reports that many devices have failed to achieve sustained user engagement.[11–13] Indeed, research on acceptance and adoption of activity trackers indicates their influence on behavior is mediated by many social, cognitive, and psychological factors, involving unique life priorities, personal circumstances, and personalities, and resulting in outcomes ranging from abandonment to strong acceptance.[11,14,15]

Thus, it has been concluded that these devices are best approached as facilitators and not drivers of behavior change in and of themselves and that their use is not one-size-fits-all. Designs and behavior change elements will continue to need to be further developed and incorporated to optimize the effect of activity trackers in promoting personal fitness that can have impact on a population level. Features such as goal-based gamification, social support, and customized output should continue to be explored in the context of the goals of the individual. The reviewed literature suggests that wearable activity trackers targeting patients with chronic illness, for example, may be most effective when integrated into programs that recommend a customized regimen and specific levels of physical activities.[11,16,17] In contrast, activity tracking targeting health office workers with sedentary behavior, as another example, may be more effective as a reminder for the user to engage in physical activity at regular intervals. Other potential solutions include alternative forms of data visualization and textual cues and designs that take users' past history into account.[11,18]

SECONDARY PREVENTION: ELECTROCARDIOGRAM DEVICES FOR EARLY DETECTION OF ATRIAL FIBRILLATION, THE MOST COMMON ARRHYTHMIA IN PEOPLE, ESPECIALLY OLDER ADULTS
Early Development

Measurement of the electrical activity of the heart is based on a relatively simple concept involving placement of electrodes on the skin at at least 2 separate points. Beginning with the first ECG machine, which was large enough to fill a room and was built in 1902 by Willem Einthoven, who a had described the wave forms of the heart's electrical activity a decade earlier, the quest to build machines of decreasing size had begun. The first portable ECG machine was developed in 1928 and weighed 20 kg. Subsequent development of transistors and ultimately microchips led to ever increasing portability.

The first wearable ECG device in the form of the Holter monitor was introduced in 1957, allowing continuous readings in ambulatory settings typically over 24 hours as a diagnostic tool. Eventually the wearable ECG would be reduced to the size of a band-aid that could be worn on the chest for up to 14 days. At the same time, devices that could be used for intermittent ECG recordings at home emerged, with AliveCor's Kardia device being one of the earliest entering the consumer market and receiving US Food and Drug Administration (FDA) approval. With the introduction of the Apple Watch and other smartwatches, this technology became truly portable, enabling ECG recordings to be recorded at the wrist by placing a finger on the electrode-containing crown of the watch.

Most of these technologies involve single lead recordings, which for many ECG uses are inferior to the 12-lead standard in medical settings. However, in both formats—continuous and intermittent recordings—they have been found accurate for detecting atrial fibrillation (AF) in comparison with the conventional 12-lead ECG. AF is an important public health target given that it is the most common arrhythmia, particularly among older adults, and its early detection and treatment are important in preventing strokes.

With the current standard of care for screening for AF being palpation to detect an irregular pulse, the use of mHealth for AF detection in fact predated the development of ECG devices. Heart rate monitoring with devices using photo-plethysmography (PPG), such as the Fitbit, led to AF detection algorithms with high sensitivity and specificity.[19] Given that ECG is the gold standard for detection of AF, the newer wrist worn ECG devices have not unexpectedly shown high sensitivity and specificity. In a meta-analysis, sensitivity of wrist worn ECG devices in individuals known to have AF was 96% overall, with a specificity among individuals in normal sinus rhythm of 98%.[20]

Devices providing continuous recordings have demonstrated even greater sensitivity, allowing detection of AF of shorter duration and lower burden, as measured as percent of time a person is in AF. In the mSToPS study involving the Zio patch, a continuous ECG device storing recordings over a 2-week period, for example, the longest episode of AF detected in individuals during a total of 2 periods (28 days) of monitoring was less than 5 minutes in 7.2% of participants, 5 minutes to 6 hours in 55%, 6 to 24 hours in 25%, and more than 24 hours in only 13% participants.[21] Numbers were similar in SCREEN-AF, another trial of continuous monitoring.[22]

Although, by definition, AF detected on ECG of any duration is AF, it is not yet clear what the associated risks of stroke with the low-duration/low-burden AF are and what the appropriate management should be (ie, what additional monitoring or what threshold for initiating treatment should be). This is a particularly important question given that treatment of AF for prevention of stroke can also come significant potential harms. Anticoagulant therapy, the primary intervention for stroke prevention, is associated with a substantial risk of bleeding, and pharmacologic, surgical, endovascular (eg, ablation), or combined treatments to control heart rhythm or heart rate can also cause harm. In addition, ECG may detect other abnormalities (either true- or false-positive results) that can lead to further testing and treatments that have further potential for harm.

The 2022 USPSTF recommendation for screening for AF reflects this uncertainty and concern for the benefit-to-harm ratio.[23,24] Noting that it considers opportunistic pulse palpation to be routine or usual care for AF detection, the task force concluded that there was currently insufficient evidence to recommend screening for AF with devices, citing that "the stroke risk associated with subclinical AF, particularly subclinical AF of shorter duration (less than several to 24 hours) or lower burden (amount or percentage of time spent in AF), as might be detected by some screening approaches, is uncertain, and the duration of subclinical AF that might warrant anticoagulant therapy is unclear."[24] Thus, the task force concluded, for the output of these devices to be truly beneficial to users as a screening tool for AF, much greater understanding of the risk of stroke associated with AF detected by these devices and that risk varies with duration and burden of AF as well as the potential benefit anticoagulation therapy among persons with subclinical AF must be demonstrated in subsequent studies.[23,24]

TERTIARY PREVENTION: CONTINUOUS GLUCOSE MONITORS FOR IMPROVED GLYCEMIC CONTROL IN PEOPLE WITH DIABETES

Glycemic control is a cornerstone of diabetes management, with the goal of preventing diabetic complications such as such as retinal, kidney and nerve damage that ultimately can result in blindness, need for dialysis, and limb amputations. Traditional methods of assessing glycemic control have been through daily self-monitoring of blood glucose (SMBG) and tracking of long-term A1C levels. Adherence to the rigid SMBG regimens required to adjust therapy, diet, and activity adequately to delay the onset and slow the progression of diabetic complications, however, is difficult, typically requiring 4 to 10 finger sticks daily. Continuous glucose monitoring (CGM) technology has been heralded as having the potential to revolutionize diabetes care by allowing greater fine-tuning of glycemic control. This is based on the idea that by providing real-time data passively collected by an implanted electrode, CGM enables more timely therapeutic interventions and changes in lifestyle or dietary intake to enhance glycemic control, with accompanying increase in quality of life because of the reduced need for finger sticks.

The basic technology underlying CGM is an enzyme-based electrode, which is inserted transdermally to measure glucose levels in interstitial fluid. Backed by extensive research and development that started in the early 1960s, the first market-able implantable glucose sensors were introduced in 1999.[25,26] These first sensors, however, proved to have limited clinical utility. They were bulky and unreliable, exhibiting significant drift in sensitivity over the initial FDA-approved 3-day implantation period, and required calibration with finger stick glucose every 6 to 12 hours. These limitations, as well as the fact that readings were not available in real time and had to be downloaded by medical professionals, diminished enthusiasm for these devices early on, and their use was relegated to primarily a supplement to SMBG.[26] In the intervening years, real-time glucose readings viewable by users on their own mobile devices with programmable high and low glucose alerts have become the state-of-the-art. Advances in sensor chemistry, sensor coatings, and improved implantation techniques have also contributed to improved biocompatibility, reducing the foreign body response and allowing extension of device lifespan from 3 days to 14 days. In the mid-2010s, flash glucose monitoring systems entered the market, allowing users to scan the receiver over the sensor to obtain their current glucose value and glucose trends and eliminated the need for repeated calibrations.

To date, uptake of the devices has been greatest among patients with type 1 diabetes, but their use among the much larger population of patients with type 2 diabetes is expected to grow rapidly. A 2021 market report estimated that of the 2.4 million CGM users in the United States at that time, up to 70% had type 1 diabetes, and only 3% to 4% of the US type 2 diabetes population was using the devices.[27] With more than 37 million persons with diabetes in the United States, growth in use is expected to increase, particularly as out-of-pocket costs–which can be hundreds of dollars per month–go down and insurance coverage increases.

RCTs comparing glycemic control with CGM versus usual care have been conducted in multiple clinical populations including persons with both type 1 and type 2 diabetes. Meta-analyses of these trials found use of CGM for periods ranging from 12 to 36 weeks was associated with modest reductions in A1C in patients with either type of diabetes, with real-time CGM leading to larger improvements in A1C compared with flash CGM.[28,29] Decreases in A1C levels in CGM versus usual care over the relatively short time periods of the studies were on the order of 0.2% to 0.3% greater for the CGM group.

Improvement in glycemic control as reflected by the decreases in A1C in participants on regimens including adjustable insulin and other therapies involved, at least in part, better fine-tuning of these therapies. However, a relatively large trial published in 2021 focused on CGM use in adults with type 2 diabetes treated only with basal insulin at baseline only and no prandial insulin showed a similar difference in mean change in A1C from baseline between CGM and usual care of −0.4% after 8 months.[30] This occurred without significant changes in amount of insulin or other treatments used, indicating that the effect involved primarily lifestyle changes in response to the glucose readings.

CGM is also providing new measures of glycemic control with the CGM-specific metric of time in range (TIR)—measured as the percent of time continuous readings are in the range of 70 to 180 mg/dL—included American Diabetes Association's recommendations for assessment of glycemic control along with A1C for tertiary prevention.[31] The document cites the association of TIR with risk of microvascular complications and published data suggesting a strong correlation between TIR and A1C as the basis of these recommendations, with a goal of 70% TIR aligning with an A1C of approximately 7%. Direct evidence of CGM's effect on long-term macrovascular outcomes is not as well established.

Continuous Glucose Monitoring in Secondary and Primary Prevention?

The findings for CGM in participants with diabetes have several implications for prevention beyond improved disease management for people with diabetes. By enabling users without diabetes to track the effects of dietary choices and physical activity on glucose levels, including spikes and prolonged periods of elevated glucose that may be triggered differently among individuals, CGM has potential for use in primary prevention of diabetes, especially among those with prediabetes. Earlier diagnosis of prediabetes and diabetes through measures such as TIR are also possible.

Beyond Continuous Glucose Monitoring: Sampling Interstitial and Other Fluids

The potential for wearable technologies involving use of electrodes to measure biochemicals in body fluids extends CGM. Sensors for DNA, for example, are being developed that will allow detection of infectious agents and cancer biomarkers applicable to all levels of preventive medicine.[32] Although the potential is also present for measurement of many other blood chemistries, it remains to be determined whether the accuracy of these methods will ever be sufficient to rival the well-established assays and efficient processes of the current system of laboratory analysis.[33]

OTHER DEVICES FOR USE TO PREVENT DISEASE AND IMPROVE HEALTH
Sleep

Activity trackers are useful not only for measuring activity, but also measuring inactivity, which in extended periods correlates with sleep. Wearing devices during sleep requires a higher level of wearability, leading to the development of rings and patches in attempt to find devices, including smart rings, that are even less obtrusive, than those worn at the wrist. Applications include primary prevention as an indicator for to promote more and better quality sleep, an important lifestyle pillar for health. Studies comparing activity tracker sleep metrics with polysomnograms have found that total sleep time and sleep efficiency are overestimated by these devices, while wake after sleep onset, an important measure of sleep quality, is underestimated.[34,35] Studies on whether availability of these data actually promote better or longer sleep are largely lacking. More sophisticated devices that integrate data including heart rate and use more sensitive motion detectors are now being used to assess time in different stages of sleep.[36] With this technology, the devices could be used in place of the polysomnogram as a diagnostic tool, allowing earlier diagnosis of sleep disorders and even for delivering the intervention. For example, these devices are being investigated for treating insomnia through sleep retraining involving repeated awakenings, as detected by the device, shortly after initiating sleep.[37–40]

Harmful Environmental Exposures

Measurement of personal exposures to environmental hazards has been another early area of mHealth, beginning with the wearing of badges to measure exposure to radiation among laboratory workers and others with potential exposures. Although these devices did not provide real-time readings, the data were actionable for primary prevention, indicating the need to limit and avoid exposures according to health guidelines. Similarly, wearable devices involving silicone wristbands combined with high throughput chemical analysis platforms capable of detecting harmful chemical exposures, including pollutants and even infectious agents, are now being developed.[41–43] The challenge with these technologies to date for quantitative exposure assessment mostly lies with the inherent complexity in calibrating them.[41]

Other Technologies on the Horizon for Health-Related Decision-Making

Devices designed to provide data for health-related decision making are also providing novel types of data not previously used in medicine, including preventive medicine. These include vocal biomarkers, including acoustic sensors for detection of cough and a smartphone-based device for detection of tonic-clonic seizures, which, combined with AI, has the ability to predict their occurrence.[33]

As reviewed by Xu and colleagues, advances are also being made in how and where sensors can be placed. Development of softer, skin-interfacing materials and continued progress in miniaturization allow placement of devices on fingernails, earlobes, and in the nose, to measure blood oxygenation and heart rate.[33] Other devices are being developed for measurement of substances in sweat and tears, including sensors in contact lenses.[33]

INTEGRATION OF MULTIPLE DEVICES/MODALITIES FOR HEALTH CARE MANAGEMENT AND PREVENTION IN PEOPLE AND POPULATIONS

While this article described the use of individual types of devices, integration of the data streams from multiple sensors representing multiple modalities holds even more promise. For example, wearable devices are part of the expansive vision of the hospital-at-home concept, wherein multiple sensors deliver data to remote patient monitoring platforms that, aided by machine learning algorithms, can guide treatment decisions by health care professionals in real time. Although the concept received a boost in interest during the coronavirus disease 2019 (COVID-19) pandemic and has been studied for use in various conditions, a recent meta-analysis reported that the use of wearables was not as common as expected in the approaches with studies published to date.[44]

Integration of multiple modalities from mHealth devices is also a concept with potential at the personal primary prevention level. One of the earliest examples of successfully using a person's "physiome" as measured by heart rate, skin temperature, blood oxygen levels, and physical activity and integrated with AI algorithms was reported by Li and colleagues in 2017,[45] demonstrating the ability to detect a Lyme disease infection before overt signs and symptoms were present. The signal prompted the individual to seek medical care and resulted in earlier diagnosis and application of effective treatment than would have been likely without the sensor data.

At the population level, aggregating multiple signals from multiple modalities from multiple people has provided a new vision of precision public health for detection of epidemics among other uses.[46–48]

Meeting Challenges in the Future

For these visions of improved personal and public health through mHealth to be realized, challenges must be addressed, including the transforming or translating of the available data to meaningful behavior changes for individuals and populations. But new technologies are also likely to incorporate solutions to this in the form of digital health coaches. Given the current state of AI, It is not hard to envision a Siri- or Alexa-style coach who is able to integrate personal health data flowing from myriad devices, prioritize actionable data, determine the most healthful responses, and interact in a personable way, answering questions like "What's the most important thing I should do for my health today?" or "How's my heart doing?" as easily as these digital assistants answer questions like "Who won the last Super Bowl?"

Another challenge that has grown along with the availability of these data is the problem of maintaining privacy, which is particularly important for health-related data. Studies have shown this to be a concern of participants in studies of biometric monitoring devices.[49] A recent article by the National Academy of Medicine underscored these concerns, arguing that transparency and consent for consumers and patients regarding data sharing, agency, and privacy within and across platforms and stakeholders must be simplified and standardized and that "privacy and security risks with big data and AI require special attention."[50]

SUMMARY

mHealth has long been available in some form, starting with activity trackers dating from the Renaissance. Modern technology has resulted in an ever-increasing number of wearable devices that can generate various health-related data. Some of the most mature of these devices to date have been successfully utilized in primary, secondary, and tertiary prevention and combinations thereof. From the examples of wearable activity trackers, ECG monitors, and CGM, the potential effects on health and the need for future research to identify and address the challenges—including the need for incorporating effective behavior change interventions, successfully integrating data from multiple sensors, and determining the long-term health effects of their use—are clear.

In the meantime, clinical use of these devices to date has been most prominent in tertiary prevention hospital-at-home settings designed to allow remote monitoring and treatment. Increased use of mHealth in combination with telemedicine can be expected as ease of use and connectivity to health systems increase, enabling further collaboration between health care providers and patients in optimizing care, including preventive care at all levels.

ACKNOWLEDGEMENT SECTION

J. Waalen was supported in part by NIH NCATS, United States grant UL1TR002550 of the Scripps Research Translational Institute.

CONFLICTS OF INTEREST STATEMENT

The author is funded as a consultant on NIH, United States/NIDDK, United States grants 1R01 DK124427-01A1. Continuous Glucose Monitoring for High-Risk Type 2 Diabetes in the Hospital: Cloud-based Real-Time Glucose Evaluation and Management System (Cyber GEMS) and R01 DK127491 Addressing Emotional Distress to Improve Outcomes among Diverse Adults with Type 1 (ACT1VATE).

REFERENCES

1. Bassett DR Jr, Toth LP, LaMunion SR, et al. Step counting: a review of measurement considerations and health-related applications. Sports Med 2017;47(7):1303–15.
2. Murakami H, Kawakami R, Nakae S, et al. Accuracy of 12 wearable devices for estimating physical activity energy expenditure using a metabolic chamber and the doubly labeled water method: validation study. JMIR Mhealth Uhealth 2019;7(8):e13938.
3. Evenson KR, Goto MM, Furberg RD. Systematic review of the validity and reliability of consumer-wearable activity trackers. Int J Behav Nutr Phys Activ 2015;12:159.
4. Fuller D, Colwell E, Low J, et al. Reliability and validity of commercially available wearable devices for measuring steps, energy expenditure, and heart rate: systematic review. JMIR Mhealth Uhealth 2020;8(9):e18694.

5. Feehan LM, Geldman J, Sayre EC, et al. Systematic review and narrative syntheses of quantitative data. JMIR Mhealth Uhealth 2018;6(8):e10527.

6. Ferguson T, Olds T, Curtis R, et al. Effectiveness of wearable activity trackers to increase physical activity and improve health: a systematic review of systematic reviews and meta-analyses. Lancet Digit Health 2022;4(8):e615–26.

7. Davergne T, Pallot A, Dechartres A, et al. Use of wearable activity trackers to improve physical activity behavior in patients with rheumatic and musculoskeletal diseases: a systematic review and meta-analysis. Arthritis Care Res 2019;71: 758–67.

8. Freak-Poli R, Cumpston M, Albarqouni L, et al. Workplace pedometer interventions for increasing physical activity. Cochrane Database Syst Rev 2020;7: CD009209.

9. Larsen RT, Christensen J, Juhl CB, et al. Physical activity monitors to enhance amount of physical activity in older adults: a systematic review and meta-analysis. Eur Rev Aging Phys Act 2019;16:7.

10. Oliveira JS, Sherrington C, Zheng ERY, et al. Effect of interventions using physical activity trackers on physical activity in people aged 60 years and over: a systematic review and meta-analysis. Br J Sports Med 2020;54:1188–94.

11. Shin G, Jarrahi MH, Fei Y, et al. Wearable activity trackers, accuracy, adoption, acceptance and health impact: a systematic literature review. J Biomed Inform 2019;93:103153.   https://linkinghub.elsevier.com/retrieve/pii/S1532-0464(19) 30071-1.

12. Dibia V. An Affective, Normative and Functional Approach to Designing User Experiences for Wearables (2015). Available at: https://doi.org/10.2139/ssrn. 2630715.

13. Meyer J., Schnauber J., Heuten W., et al., "Exploring Longitudinal Use of Activity Trackers," 2016 IEEE International Conference on Healthcare Informatics (ICHI), Chicago, IL, USA, 2016, pp. 198-206. https://doi.org/10.1109/ICHI.2016.29.

14. Jarrahi MH, Gafinowitz N, Shin G. Activity trackers, prior motivation, and perceived informational and motivational affordances 2018;22:433–48.

15. Jarrahi MH, Nelson SB, Thomson L. Personal artifact ecologies in the context of mobile knowledge workers. Comput Hum Behav 2017;75:469–83.

16. Mercer K, Giangregorio L, Schneider E, et al. Acceptance of commercially available wearable activity trackers among adults aged over 50 and with chronic illness: a mixed-methods evaluation. JMIR mHealth and uHealth 2016;4(1):e7.

17. Mercer K, Li M, Giangregorio L, et al. Behavior change techniques present in wearable activity trackers: a critical analysis. JMIR mHealth and uHealth 2016; 4(2):e4.

18. Epstein DA, Kang JH, Pina LR, et al. Reconsidering the Device in the Drawer: Lapses as a Design Opportunity in Personal Informatics. Proc ACM Int Conf Ubiquitous Comput 2016;2016:829–40.

19. Hochstadt A, Chorin E, Viskin S, et al. Continuous heart rate monitoring for automatic detection of atrial fibrillation with novel bio-sensing technology. J Electrocardiol 2019;52:23–7.

20. Belani S, Wahood W, Hardigan P, et al. Accuracy of detecting atrial fibrillation: a systematic review and meta-analysis of wrist-worn wearable technology. Cureus 2021;13(12):e20362.

21. Steinhubl SR, Waalen J, Edwards AM, et al. Effect of a home-based wearable continuous ecg monitoring patch on detection of undiagnosed atrial fibrillation: the mSToPS randomized clinical trial. JAMA 2018;320(2):146–55.

22. Gladstone DJ, Wachter R, Schmalstieg-Bahr K, et al. Screening for atrial fibrillation in the older population: a randomized clinical trial. JAMA Cardiol 2021;6(5): 558–67.

23. US Preventive Services Task Force, Davidson KW, Barry MJ, et al. Screening for atrial fibrillation: US preventive services task force recommendation statement. JAMA 2022;327(4):360–7.

24. Kahwati LC, Asher GN, Kadro ZO, et al. Screening for atrial fibrillation: updated evidence report and systematic review for the US preventive services task force. JAMA 2022;327(4):368–83.

25. Papanikolaou E, Simos YV, Spyrou K, et al. Is graphene the rock upon which new era continuous glucose monitors could be built? Exp Biol Med 2023;248(1): 14–25.

26. Didyuk O, Econom N, Guardia A, et al. Continuous glucose monitoring devices: past, present, and future focus on the history and evolution of technological innovation. J Diabetes Sci Technol 2021;15(3):676–83.

27. Available at: https://www.diabetesdata.org/cgm-data/accessed. Accessed April 11, 2023.

28. Di Molfetta S, Caruso I, Cignarelli A, et al. Professional continuous glucose monitoring in patients with diabetes mellitus: a systematic review and meta-analysis. Diabetes Obes Metab 2023;25(5):1301–10.

29. Maiorino MI, Signoriello S, Maio A, et al. Effects of continuous glucose monitoring on metrics of glycemic control in diabetes: a systematic review with meta-analysis of randomized controlled trials. Diabetes Care 2020;43(5):1146–56.

30. Martens T, Beck RW, Bailey R, et al. Effect of continuous glucose monitoring on glycemic control in patients with type 2 diabetes treated with basal insulin: a randomized clinical trial. JAMA 2021;325(22):2262–72.

31. American Diabetes Association Professional Practice Committee; 6. Glycemic targets: standards of medical care in diabetes—2022. Diabetes Care 2022;45(Suppl_1). S83 96.

32. Biswas GC, Khan MTM, Das J. Wearable nucleic acid testing platform - a perspective on rapid self-diagnosis and surveillance of infectious diseases. Biosens Bioelectron 2023;226:115115.

33. Xu S, Kim J, Walter JR, et al. Translational gaps and opportunities for medical wearables in digital health. Sci Transl Med 2022;14(666):eabn6036.

34. Evenson KR, Goto MM, Furburg RD. Systematic review of the validity and reliability of consumer-wearable activity trackers. Int J Behav Nutr Phys Activ 2015;12:159.

35. de Zambotti M, Cellini N, Goldstone A, et al. Wearable sleep technology in clinical and research settings. Med Sci Sports Exerc 2019;51(7):1538–57.

36. Menghini L, Yuksel D, Goldstone A, et al. Performance of Fitbit Charge 3 against polysomnography in measuring sleep in adolescent boys and girls. Chronobiol Int 2021;38(7):1010–22.

37. Lai MYC, Mong MSA, Cheng LJ, et al. The effect of wearable-delivered sleep interventions on sleep outcomes among adults: a systematic review and meta-analysis of randomized controlled trials. Nurs Health Sci 2022. https://doi.org/10.1111/nhs.13011.

38. Scott H, Lechat B, Manners J, et al. Emerging applications of objective sleep assessments towards the improved management of insomnia. Sleep Med 2023; 101:138–45.

39. Bensen-Boakes DB, Murali T, Lovato N, et al. Wearable device-delivered intensive sleep retraining as an adjunctive treatment to kickstart cognitive-behavioral therapy for insomnia. Sleep Med Clin 2023;18(1):49–57.

40. Aji M, Glozier N, Bartlett DJ, et al. The effectiveness of digital insomnia treatment with adjunctive wearable technology: a pilot randomized controlled trial. Behav Sleep Med 2022;20(5):570–83.

41. Okeme JO, Koelmel JP, Johnson E, et al. Wearable passive samplers for assessing environmental exposure to organic chemicals: current approaches and future directions. Curr Environ Health Rep 2023. https://doi.org/10.1007/s40572-023-00392-w.

42. Guo P, Lin EZ, Koelmel JP, et al. Exploring personal chemical exposures in China with wearable air pollutant monitors: a repeated-measure study in healthy older adults in Jinan, China. Environ Int 2021;156:106709.

43. Koelmel JP, Lin EZ, Nichols A, et al. Head, shoulders, knees, and toes: placement of wearable passive samplers alters exposure profiles observed. Environ Sci Technol 2021;55(6):3796–806.

44. Denecke K, May R, Borycki EM, et al. Digital health as an enabler for hospital@home: a rising trend or just a vision? Front Public Health 2023;11:1137798.

45. Li X, Dunn J, Salins D, et al. Digital health: tracking physiomes and activity using wearable biosensors reveals useful health-related information. PLoS Biol 2017; 15(1):e2001402.

46. Alavi A, Bogu GK, Wang M, et al. Real-time alerting system for COVID-19 and other stress events using wearable data. Nat Med 2022;28(1):175–84.

47. Gadaleta M, Radin JM, Baca-Motes K, et al. Passive detection of COVID-19 with wearable sensors and explainable machine learning algorithms. NPJ Digit Med 2021;4(1):166.

48. Radin JM, Quer G, Pandit JA, et al. Sensor-based surveillance for digitising real-time COVID-19 tracking in the USA (DETECT): a multivariable, population-based, modelling study. Lancet Digit Health 2022;4(11):e777–86.

49. Perlmutter A, Benchoufi M, Ravaud P, et al. Identification of patient perceptions that can affect the uptake of interventions using biometric monitoring devices: systematic review of randomized controlled trials. J Med Internet Res 2020; 22(9):e18986.

50. Abernethy A, Adams L, Barrett M, et al. The promise of digital health: then, now, and the future. NAM Perspectives. Washington, DC: Discussion paper, National Academy of Medicine; 2022.

Lifestyle Medicine
Prevention, Treatment, and Reversal of Disease

Michael D. Parkinson, MD, MPH, FACPM[a],*, Ron Stout, MD, MPH[b],
Wayne Dysinger, MD, MPH[c]

KEYWORDS

- Lifestyle medicine • Health behaviors • Medical curriculum • Preventive medicine
- Whole person health • Chronic disease • Population health • Reimbursement

KEY POINTS

- Lifestyle medicine (LM) focuses on six pillars—a plant-predominant eating pattern; physical movement; restorative sleep; management of stress; avoidance of risky substances; and positive social connections.
- LM expands the scope of preventive medicine by focusing on the promotion of healthy lifestyles while preventing, treating, and reversing the majority of chronic diseases.
- Whole health care is an interprofessional, team-based approach anchored in trusted relationships to promote well-being, prevent disease, and restore health.

HISTORY AND BACKGROUND

The actual causes of death in the United States were first articulated in a landmark 1993 analysis by Dr. Michael McGinnis of the Federal Office of Disease Prevention and Health Promotion and Dr. Bill Foege of the Centers for Disease Control.[1] The study, updated in the early 2000s, demonstrated that personal health behaviors, and the environmental factors promoting or impeding them, remained the most significant contributors to mortality.[2] Lifestyle behaviors such as tobacco use, poor diet, physical inactivity, and excessive alcohol use are the primary causes of chronic diseases leading to premature deaths. Despite this evidence, physicians have not routinely or systematically received the education, training, practice skills, and support to address these root cause behavioral and environmental challenges faced by patients.

Responding to this ongoing deficit and the growing demand by physicians for training and recognition in promoting effective patient behavior change, the American College of Preventive Medicine (ACPM) hosted the Blue Ribbon Panel on Lifestyle

[a] P3 Health, LLC (Prevention, Performance, Productivity), 5864 Aylesboro Avenue, Pittsburgh, PA 15217, USA; [b] Ardmore Institute of Health, PO Box 1269, Ardmore, OK 73402, USA; [c] Lifestyle Medical, 4368 Central Avenue, Riverside, CA 92506, USA
* Corresponding author.
E-mail address: mdparkinson14@gmail.com

Med Clin N Am 107 (2023) 1109–1120
https://doi.org/10.1016/j.mcna.2023.06.007
0025-7125/23/© 2023 Elsevier Inc. All rights reserved.

Medicine Competency Development in 2009.[3] Representatives of all major medical primary care and related specialty societies defined physician competencies in five essential and mutually-reinforcing domains: leadership, knowledge, assessment skills, management skills, and use of office and community support. These physician and practice competencies represented a foundational building block for undergraduate and graduate medical students, practicing physicians, health professionals, and health systems to not only prevent but also treat and even reverse most chronic diseases.

The rapid growth of lifestyle medicine (LM) and expanding interest by health practitioners led to the LM core competencies being updated in 2022, expanding from 15 to 88 competencies and 5 to 10 domains.[4] The focus now includes the science of LM, leadership and advocacy, nutrition, physical activity, sleep hygiene, risky substances, clinical processes, health behavior change, emotional and mental health, connectedness, and positive psychology.

Scientific and Clinical Practice Evidence Supporting LM

The nearly 70-year-old medical specialty of preventive medicine has been rooted in the evidence that both public health and the clinical practice of prevention in medical care are essential for disease prevention and health promotion.[5] Primary prevention (health promotion, immunizations), secondary prevention (early detection, screening, and case finding), and tertiary prevention (prevention of disease progression through treatment) represent a continuum long recognized by the field of preventive medicine.

The groundbreaking work of the U.S. Preventive Services Task Force (USPSTF) first published in 1989 codified the evidence hierarchy for evaluation of the periodic health examination and the importance of delivering age, gender, and risk-specific screening tests, counseling, and immunizations.[6] These primary and secondary preventive services rely on providers being competent in delivering them and on creating a supportive clinic practice ecosystem. The specialty of preventive medicine embraced clinical preventive medicine to advance the optimal delivery of evidence-based services based on the USPSTF recommendations. However, the USPSTF did not include the *treatment* (tertiary prevention) of existing diseases or conditions in its charge and neither did the practice of "clinical preventive medicine" in its scope or goals.

At the same time, clinical evidence of the impact of lifestyle changes on disease treatment and reversal was growing. Drs. Dean Ornish and Caldwell Esselstyn, among others, demonstrated that lifestyle interventions with a focus on whole food plant-based eating, physical activity, and stress reduction could prevent the progression of atherosclerotic cardiovascular disease, the recurrence of cardiac events, and even reverse angiographically observed coronary artery plaque.[7,8]

Advances in basic science understanding of epigenetics, microbiome, neuroplasticity, and cellular function reinforced that lifestyle behaviors had a direct impact on the causation and reversal of common disease processes. Physicians from multiple specialties began to articulate the urgent need for prioritizing LM in the treatment of leading causes of disease producing premature morbidity and mortality.[9]

The continued rise in the burden of chronic disease not only in the United States but worldwide, the underfunding of prevention research particularly relating to lifestyle behaviors in disease treatment[10] and the growing body of basic science and clinical practice data lead to the convening of the Lifestyle Medicine Research Summit in 2019.[11] Fifty nationally recognized expert basic science and clinical researchers and practitioners reviewed the evidence for each of the six pillars of LM—plant-based eating pattern, physical activity, restorative sleep, stress management, avoidance of risky substances, and positive social connections, in preventing, treating, and reversing common chronic and other diseases. **Fig. 1** captures the major conclusions of the summit, demonstrating the common causal pathway of systemic chronic inflammation leading to disease and disease progression which can be initiated, promoted, or reversed through lifestyle interventions.

The summit also intensely discussed and summarized the role of social determinants of health (SDoH) influences, environment, and exposures, particularly in the context of underserved and understudied populations which historically suffer a disproportionate disease burden increasingly being linked to impactful inequities and disparities. Toxic stress in early childhood from psychological trauma, physical abuse or adverse childhood experiences, environmental chemical exposures, and low-grade chronic inflammation caused by systemic racism is known to affect neurologic development and increase the risk of medical and psychological chronic diseases.[12,13] Research priorities for the six LM domains included recommendations for focused explorations of the impact of culturally sensitive and demographically tailored approaches to address lifestyle and environmental challenges in disadvantaged populations and geographies.

LM Competent Physicians and Practices

Multiple foundational changes need to be realized in order for LM to make a measurable difference in health, health care outcomes and health care systems. Health care professionals need a basic understanding of the six LM pillars and their primary role(s) in addressing the root causes and solutions in disease prevention, treatment, and

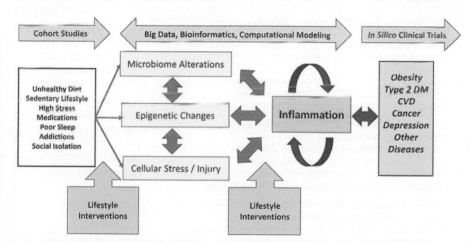

Fig. 1. Lifestyle-associated pathogeniesis, interventions, and emerging methods for lifestyle medicine research. [a]Lifestyle-associated pathogeniesis, interventions, and emerging methods for lifestyle medicine research. Unhealthy lifestyles cause dysergulation in the microbiome, epigenetic changes, and various types of cellular stress and injury which, together, drive inflammation. In turn, inflammation can drive further derangements in the microbiome, can cause distinct epigenetic changes, and can drive further cellular stress and injury. This positive feedback leads to a process wherein inflammation becomes chronic and self-sustaining, ultimately resulting in chronic diseases, such as Type 2 diabetes. The non-linear nature of these processes means that they fail. Effective lifestyle interventions prevent, treat, and reverse common chronic diseases. To accelerate the adoption and dissemination of clinical lifestyle medicine interventions, there is a need for cutting-edge biological and computational approaches to decipher this complexity. ([a]*From* Frontiers in Medicine,[11] with permission. Available via Creative Commons CC-BY license, Version 4.0.)

reversal. In addition, a holistic LM primary care approach is fundamentally different from the traditional reductionistic allopathic medicine models. Differences include team-based care, group sessions, practice setting alterations, preferred reimbursement models,[14,15] and the creation and inclusion of an LM intensivist within health systems.[16] Intensivists can adjust patient medications, lead patient group sessions, and provide treatment using Intensive Therapeutic Lifestyle Change.[17] The American Board of Lifestyle Medicine (ABLM) created experiential and educational pathways qualifying for separate certification as an LM Intensivist.[18]

LM in Primary Care Practice

An example of LM in the clinical practice is the Holistic LM Primary care model,[19] which has four organizing components (**Box 1**).

- Foundational Concepts: Open Heart, Deep Caring. The provider connects with the patient "heart to heart" demonstrating "deep caring" and "family-level commitment." Providers explore details of a patient's life, including family and friend networks, living situations, occupations, and vocations.
- Assessment Approaches: Antecedents and Triggers. Antecedents include genetic and environmental experiences that affect how someone operates.[22] Triggers are day-to-day exposures resulting in hindbrain survival approaches that are counterproductive to achieving optimal health. These are explored through unique vital signs and comprehensive assessments.

Box 1
Holistic Lifestyle Medicine Primary Care Components[15,20,21]

Foundational Concepts: Open Heart, Deep Caring Attitude
- Relaxing "spa-like" clinic atmosphere
- Extended visits
- Capitated or membership reimbursement model
- Board-certified providers in lifestyle medicine
- Medical assistants with additional training in health coaching and empathy

Assessment Approaches: Antecedents and Triggers
- Lifestyle medicine vital signs at every visit
  - Subjective 30-second check of the LM pillars
- Nutrition assessments[20] initially and annually
- Lifestyle medicine comprehensive physical activity assessment[21] initially and annually
- Electronic medical record sections for each LM pillar

Treatment Approaches: Implementing Behavior Change
- Lifestyle medicine clinical protocols
- Customizable lifestyle medicine prescription templates
- A team available to assist in achieving health goals includes a registered dietitian, personal trainer, social worker, certified wellness coach, occupational therapist, and others.
- Groups visits
  - Weekly in-person and virtual support groups including nutrition, exercise, meditation, and health behavior change groups
  - Periodic cooking classes, walk with the doctor events, and other resources

Maintenance Approaches: Staying Connected
- Documentation of social connections
- Regular provider communication availability through either the electronic medical record or an interactive patient app
- Same-day acute or within one-week semi-acute appointments
- Proactive tracking of health risks and connecting with patients at an appropriate frequency based on the health risk profile

- Treatment Approaches: Implementing Behavior Change. Positive psychology builds on the strengths and affirming experiences of the patient, while motivational interviewing honors the concept that patients effectively come to their own best path forward. This is facilitated through the use of LM prescriptions, protocols, groups, and team resources.
- Maintenance Approaches: Staying Connected. Periodic follow-up and reinforcement for sustained behavior change.

Reimbursement Models for LM

Traditional health care reimbursement models focus on a fee-for-service model which incentivizes sick care. The ACLM has created resources to assist practices in approaching reimbursement from this perspective.[23] A more effective model for LM is a capitated or membership model whereby a periodic fee is paid by the patient, employer, or insurer. The capitated model economically motivates the holistic LM primary care provider to keep the patient healthy and reduce the total cost of care.

Opportunities for capitated reimbursement are currently best captured in the Medicare Advantage (or HMO Medicare) reimbursement model.[24] Medicare also created the Accountable Care Organization Realizing Equity, Access and Community Health (ACO REACH) for original and PPO Medicare recipients, providing contracted providers the ability to be reimbursed in a capitated fashion. A capitated reimbursement system using LM approaches has also been introduced for employers, through whom most Americans obtain their health insurance.[25] The Direct primary care approach is another growing subscription-based model that provides patients unlimited access to a care provider with an established monthly fee.[26]

Measurement of health care quality is frequently assessed using a triple aim approach[27] (**Fig. 2**). Early reported experience from a primary care practice specifically developed using a holistic LM model has shown improvement in all three domains.[28] The LM practice operates under a capitated or value-based care payment model and has shown preliminary positive improvement in each of the triple aim goals:

Patient clinical outcomes showed a 20% reduction in low-density lipoprotein cholesterol, a 12% reduction in HgbA1C, and a 9% reduction in body mass index

Lifestyle Medical Triple Aim Outcomes Data

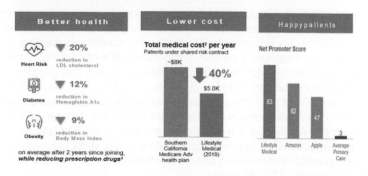

Fig. 2. Triple aim measurements and outcomes. (*Data from* Dysinger, W. Lifestyle Medical Clinic:internal practice data. Riverside, CA; 2019.)

(based on data from 55 patients over 2 years who joined the practice with elevated measures).

Patient satisfaction showed a net promoter score (NPS) average of 83 (based on NPS surveys sent to a revolving selected patient sample from a 1211 patient cohort on a monthly basis). This is compared to a typical primary care practice with an average NPS of 3.

Health care costs showed an average of $3000 annual cost savings compared to regional Medicare Advantage mean patient costs representing a 40% decrease over 3 years (based on 102 Medicare Advantage patients). Although promising, the data are preliminary, and ongoing research is needed to demonstrate significant and sustained improvements in clinical outcomes, patient satisfaction, and cost.

LM Education and Resources

Over the last 10 years, an increasing number of medical schools offer LM as part of the curriculum. The University of South Carolina School of Medicine Greenville was the first medical school in the United States to include a 4-year LM curriculum.[29] The program's focus is to promote student self-care in the areas of nutrition, physical activity, behavior change, and resiliency while preparing them with the knowledge, skills, and advocacy to support their future patients. They also launched Lifestyle Medicine Education as an open-access evidence-based LM curricular resource for medical students. Another example of an LM program is the *Health Meets Food* Culinary Medicine comprehensive training program utilized at over 60 medical schools.[30] The program increases competencies and conversations about food and lifestyle between health care providers and patients.

Medical residency programs have also expanded their curriculum to include LM training. In 2022, the Lifestyle Medicine Residency Curriculum (LMRC) was included in over 170 programs in the United States, the majority being family practice.[31] LMRC consists of a 100-hour educational component, including didactic units and independent application activities, followed by a practical experience.[32] In 2017, LM certification became available from the ABLM for physicians and health care providers.[33] ABLM diplomate certification signifies specialized LM knowledge and competencies. To date, approximately 2500 US physicians have been certified.

ACPM Support for LM

In 2017, ACPM introduced an American Medical Association proposal supporting policies and mechanisms that incentivize and provide funding for the inclusion of LM education and SDoH in undergraduate, graduate, and continuing medical education (CME).[34] LM training began as a partnership between ACPM and the American College of Lifestyle Medicine (ACLM). With over 8000 members and growing, ACLM is a medical professional society whose aim is "to provide quality education to those dedicated to clinical and worksite practice of LM as the foundation of a transformed and sustainable health care system."[35] This partnership produced the LM training program titled *Lifestyle Medicine Core Competencies*, now in its third update.[36] The 10-module program focuses on improving competence and skills, encourages a team approach, and provides the research and clinical foundation for the field. Available online, the course awards 32 CME credits.

Finally, a recent consensus statement, *Lifestyle Medicine for Optimal Outcomes in Primary Care,*[37] provides the evidence-based essential elements of an LM competent primary care practice. Physicians looking to incorporate LM into their health care practice can begin by exploring publicly available resources.[38] Additional resources to engage and educate patients include ACLM certified programs—both fee and free programs are available.[39]

Growing Synergies of Preventive Medicine, Public Health, and LM

There is growing congruence between preventive and LM, whole person health, integrative, culinary, and complementary medicine. Examples include the National Institutes of Health's National Center for Complementary and Integrative Health focus on whole person health[40] and the Veterans Health Administration Whole Health transformation effort.[41] Whole health is a team-based approach based on trusted relationships to promote well-being, prevent disease, and restore health. This approach empowers individuals, families, communities, and populations to improve their health by utilizing self-care, lifestyle, and behavioral interventions.

Momentum for LM increased in late 2022 with the White House Conference on Hunger, Nutrition, and Health. The conference laid out a vision for ending hunger and reducing diet-related disease by 2030, while closing disparities among the communities that are impacted most.[42] In collaboration with the conference, ACLM created opportunities for LM continuing education[43] by providing an online CME at no cost. ACLM and ABLM also created support for LM training and certification in each U.S. Federally Qualified Health Center in the U.S.[44]

COVID Lessons Learned and the Future ahead

In 2019, two global pandemics—COVID-19 and obesity—intersected, exacerbating the virus' most harmful effects and disproportionately affecting underserved communities. To a large extent, the underlying health conditions, that heightened vulnerability to the virus, are lifestyle-related and directly impacted by SDoH. These unhealthy lifestyle behaviors increasingly affect health care expenditure, driving as much as 90% of health care dollars spent, making the precepts of LM more relevant and more urgently needed than ever.[45] The COVID-19 pandemic and a heightened awareness of systemic racism in the health care system give a sense of urgency to increase health equity and reduce the prevalence of preventable noncommunicable diseases such as hypertension and diabetes, particularly among higher-risk populations. In order to advance these precepts, the ACPM, in late 2020, convened a group of 24 stakeholders representing leading national health care organizations and collectively articulated recommendations for integrating lifestyle and preventive medicine contents into undergraduate medical education (UME).[46] The assumption is that integrating the contents of lifestyle and preventive medicine into UME will result in content and curriculum that is better aligned with population health needs and train physicians to be better equipped to meet future demands.

Recognizing continuing gaps in medical education, the Association of American Medical Colleges and the Accreditation Council for Graduate Medical Education committed to hosting the Medical Education Summit on Nutrition in Practice in March 2023,[47] bringing together over 150 leaders in medical education to explore the best approaches for integrating nutrition and food insecurity into medical education, with a focus on interprofessional treatment and health equity.

Virtual Practices

LM can be delivered via a wide variety of standard and multimedia formats targeted to different learning styles, thus improving patient engagement and health outcomes. There is sufficient evidence to support the use of many current technologies in the clinical practice of LM.[48] During the pandemic, patient satisfaction and efficacy were demonstrated when a weight-management clinic rapidly converted to telephone appointments while maintaining close interdisciplinary collaboration.[49]

The COVID-19 pandemic expedited the utilization and acceptance of both individual and shared medical appointment (SMA) telehealth encounters. As early as 2010, virtual Complete Health Improvement Program SMAs were piloted in an employee population, with financial metrics demonstrating a return of $1.8 for every $1 invested. Requiring little physical space, virtual SMAs create an opportunity for greater scheduling flexibility while offering new opportunities for LM education and the involvement of other family members.[50]

Integration of Public Health, Preventive and LM: Whole Health

After COVID's peak, much has been written about weak public health infrastructure, lack of commitment to preventive medicine, and a significant need for greater investment. America should be committed to a community-based, equity-focused approach that optimizes well-being. A vision and strategy that educates, enables, and engages individuals within their communities combining historical and emerging practice frameworks are needed to address the conditions that enabled the inequitably distributed morbidity and mortality exacerbated by COVID. Through its Health Equity Achieved through Lifestyle Medicine (HEAL) project,[51] ACLM convened researchers, health care professionals, clergy, and community leaders. Participants concluded that now is the time to identify and eradicate the root causes of the chronic diseases, which disproportionately impact underserved communities. The consensus was that LM is a critical component and foundation of a transformed and sustainable system of health care.[52]

LM reframes the challenge of simply treating disease to recognizing, educating, and supporting patients' healthy and disease-reversing behaviors in their contextual environment, comprehensively addressing root causes. The National Academy of Medicine[53] boldly summarized the need to change the way we care for Americans: "Whole health is physical, behavioral, spiritual, and socioeconomic well-being as defined by individuals, families, and communities. Whole health care is an interprofessional, team-based approach anchored in trusted relationships to promote well-being, prevent disease, and restore health. It aligns with a person's life mission, aspiration, and purpose. It shifts the focus from a reactive disease-oriented medical care system to one that prioritizes health, well-being, and disease prevention. It changes the health care conversation from "What's wrong with you?" to "What matters to you?""

CLINICS CARE POINTS

- Lifestyle medicine (LM) clinical practice directly addresses and decreases systemic inflammation which is the common pathogenic pathway causing the majority of chronic diseases.

- LM honors the patient's beliefs and desires, collects "lifestyle vital signs", and creates a provider-patient plan and ongoing support for sustained behavior change.

- LM is optimized with aligned payment models; team-based care; skill-building; and individual, group, virtual visits and connectivity.

DISCLOSURE

Dr Parkinson is the Principal of P3 Health, LLC. Dr Parkinson serves on numerous boards and committees related to lifestyle medicine. Dr. Stout is the President &

CEO of Ardmore Institute of Health, a non-profit and active proponent of lifestyle medicine, including the provision of funding for research and publications related to lifestyle medicine. Dr. Stout serves on numerous boards and committees related to lifestyle medicine. Dr Dysinger is the CEO of Lifestyle Medical, a corporation that provides lifestyle medicine services. Dr Dysinger serves on numerous boards and committees related to lifestyle medicine.

REFERENCES

1. McGinnis JM, Foege WH. Actual causes of death in the United States. JAMA 1993;270(18):2207–12.
2. Mokdad AH, Marks JS, Stroup DF, et al. Correction: actual causes of death in the United States, 2000. JAMA 2005;293(3):293–4.
3. Lianov L, Johnson M. Physician competencies for prescribing lifestyle medicine. JAMA 2010;304(2):202–3.
4. Lianov LS, Adamson K, Kelly JH, et al. Lifestyle medicine core competencies: 2022 update. Am J Lifestyle Med 2022;16(6):734–9.
5. Ring AR. History of the American board of preventive medicine. Am J Prev Med 2002;22(4):296–319.
6. U.S. Preventive Services Task Force. Guide to Clinical Preventive Services: An Assessment of the Effectiveness of 169 Interventions : Report of the U.s. Preventive Services Task Force.; 1989.
7. Ornish D, Scherwitz LW, Billings JH, et al. Intensive lifestyle changes for reversal of coronary heart disease. JAMA 1998;280(23):2001–7.
8. Esselstyn CB Jr, Gendy G, Doyle J, et al. A way to reverse CAD? J Fam Pract 2014;63(7):356–364b.
9. Bodai B. Lifestyle medicine: A brief review of its dramatic impact on health and survival. Perm J 2017;22(1). https://doi.org/10.7812/tpp/17-025.
10. Vargas AJ, Schully SD, Villani J, et al. Assessment of prevention research measuring leading risk factors and causes of mortality and disability supported by the US National Institutes of health. JAMA Netw Open 2019;2(11):e1914718.
11. Vodovotz Y, Barnard N, Hu FB, et al. Prioritized research for the prevention, treatment, and reversal of chronic disease: Recommendations from the Lifestyle Medicine Research Summit. Front Med 2020;7:585744.
12. Shonkoff JP, Boyce WT, McEwen BS. Neuroscience, molecular biology, and the childhood roots of health disparities: building a new framework for health promotion and disease prevention: Building a new framework for health promotion and disease prevention. JAMA 2009;301(21):2252–9.
13. Lippard ETC, Nemeroff CB. The devastating clinical consequences of child abuse and neglect: Increased disease vulnerability and poor treatment response in mood disorders. Am J Psychiatry 2020;177(1):20–36.
14. Bharati R, Kovach KA, Bonnet JP. Incorporating Lifestyle Medicine Into Primary Care Practice: Perceptions and Practices of Family Physicians. Am J Lifestyle Med 2022;(0). https://doi.org/10.1177/15598276211072506.
15. Dysinger WS. A hybrid value-based lifestyle medicine practice model. Am J Lifestyle Med 2021;15(5):553–4.
16. Kelly J, Karlsen MC, Lianov L. Establishing competencies for physicians who specialize in the practice of lifestyle medicine. Am J Lifestyle Med 2020;14(2):150–4.
17. Mechley A, Dysinger W. Intensive Therapeutic Lifestyle Change Programs: A Progressive Way to Successfully Manage Health Care. Am J Lifestyle Med 2015;9(5).

18. Lifestyle medicine certification. American Board of Lifestyle Medicine. Published November 8, 2022. https://ablm.org/lifestyle-medicine-certification. Accessed January 22, 2023.

19. Dysinger W. Restore your whole health. Lifestyle Medical 2019. Available at: https://lifestylemedical.com. Accessed February 14, 2023.

20. Katz DL, Rhee LQ, Katz CS, et al. Dietary assessment can be based on pattern recognition rather than recall. Med Hypotheses 2020;140:109644.

21. Young J, Bonnet JP, Sokolof J. Lifestyle Medicine: Physical Activity. J Fam Pract 2022;71(Suppl 1 Lifestyle):S17–23.

22. Petruccelli K, Davis J, Berman T. Adverse childhood experiences and associated health outcomes: A systematic review and meta-analysis. Child Abuse Negl 2019;97(104127):104127.

23. Gobble J, Donohue D, Grega M. Reimbursement as a catalyst for advancing lifestyle medicine practices. J Fam Pract 2022;71(Suppl 1 Lifestyle):eS105–9.

24. Cubanski J, Neuman T. What to know about Medicare spending and financing. KFF. Published January 19, 2023. https://www.kff.org/medicare/issue-brief/what-to-know-about-medicare-spending-and-financing. Accessed January 14, 2023.

25. Gulati M, Delaney M. The lifestyle medicine physician's case to self-insured employers: A business model for physicians, a bargain for companies. Am J Lifestyle Med 2019;13(5):462–9.

26. Brekke G, Onge JS, Kimminau K, et al. Direct primary care: Family physician perceptions of a growing model. Popul Med 2021;3(August):1–8.

27. Berwick DM, Nolan TW, Whittington J. The triple aim: care, health, and cost. Health Aff 2008;27(3):759–69.

28. Dysinger, W. A hybrid value based lifestyle medicine practice. Presented at the American College of Lifestyle Medicine Annual Conference. October 23, 2020. Virtual.

29. Trilk JL, Muscato D, Polak R. Advancing lifestyle medicine education in undergraduate medical school curricula through the Lifestyle Medicine Education Collaborative (LMEd). Am J Lifestyle Med 2018;12(5):412–8.

30. Magallanes E, Sen A, Siler M, et al. Nutrition from the kitchen: culinary medicine impacts students' counseling confidence. BMC Med Educ 2021;21(1):88.

31. American College of Lifestyle Medicine. LMRC current sites and programs. Lifestylemedicine.org. https://lifestylemedicine.org/wp-content/uploads/2022/12/LMRC-Sites-and-Programs-2022.pdf. Accessed February 14, 2023.

32. Trilk JL, Worthman S, Shetty P, et al. Undergraduate medical education: Lifestyle Medicine curriculum implementation standards. Am J Lifestyle Med 2021;15(5):526–30.

33. Rosenfeld RM. Physician Attitudes on the Status, Value, and Future of Board Certification in Lifestyle Medicine. Am J Lifestyle Med 2022;(0). https://doi.org/10.1177/15598276221131524.

34. Trilk J, Nelson L, Briggs A, et al. Including lifestyle medicine in medical education: Rationale for American College of Preventive Medicine/American medical association Resolution 959. Am J Prev Med 2019;56(5):e169–75.

35. Rippe JM. American journal of lifestyle medicine 2023: Continued progress, enormous national and international implications. Am J Lifestyle Med 2023;17(1):5–7.

36. American College of Lifestyle Medicine. Lifestyle medicine core competencies program. Acpm.org. https://www.acpm.org/education-events/continuing-medical-education/2019/lifestyle-medicine-core-competencies-program/. Accessed January 24, 2023.

37. Lifestyle medicine for optimal outcomes in primary care. Am J Lifestyle Med 2023. Forthcoming Publication.

38. Lifestyle medicine resources for clinicians. Ardmore Institute of Health. https://www.ardmoreinstituteofhealth.org/lifestyle-medicine-resources-clinicians. Accessed March 4, 2023.

39. American College of Lifestyle Medicine. Lifestyle Medicine programs certified by ACLM. Lifestylemedicine.org. Accessed February 14, 2023. Available at: https://lifestylemedicine.org/certified-programs/.

40. National Center for Complementary and Integrative Medicine. NCCIH strategic plan FY 2021–2025. Accessed February 4, 2023. Available at: https://www.nccih.nih.gov/about/nccih-strategic-plan-2021-2025.

41. Krejci LP, Carter K, Gaudet T. Whole health: The vision and implementation of personalized, proactive, patient-driven health care for veterans. Med Care 2014;52(Supplement 5):S5–8.

42. Office of Disease Prevention and Health Promotion. White House Conference on Hunger, Nutrition, and Health. Available at: https://health.gov/our-work/nutrition-physical-activity/white-house-conference-hunger-nutrition-and-health/conference-details.

43. American College of Lifestyle Medicine. Lifestyle Medicine & Food as Medicine Essentials Bundle. Lifestylemedicine.org 2022;. http://www.lifestylemedicine.org/WHConference. Accessed February 14, 2023.

44. American College of Lifestyle Medicine. White House spotlights $24.1 million commitment by The American College of Lifestyle Medicine to advance physician and other clinician training in food as medicine to address epidemic of diet-related chronic disease. PR Newswire. Published September 28, 2022. Accessed January 24, 2023. Available at: https://www.prnewswire.com/news-releases/white-house-spotlights-24-1-million-commitment-by-the-american-college-of-lifestyle-medicine-to-advance-physician-and-other-clinician-training-in-food-as-medicine-to-address-epidemic-of-diet-related-chronic-disease-301635076.html.

45. American College of Lifestyle Medicine. A family physician's introduction to lifestyle medicine. Supplement to The Journal of Family Practice 2022;71(1):S1–72.

46. American College of Preventive Medicine. Strategic roadmap for integrating lifestyle and preventive medicine into undergraduate medical education. Acpm.org. Available at: https://www.acpm.org/media/documents/acpm-white-paper_strategic-roadmap-for-integrating-lifestyle-and-preventive-medicine-into-ume_final.pdf. Accessed January 24, 2023.

47. Frieden J. Clinicians need more training in nutrition education and spotting hunger, Biden says. MedpageToday. Published September 28, 2022. Available at: https://www.medpagetoday.com/primarycare/dietnutrition/100961. Accessed February 24, 2023.

48. Lacagnina S, Tips J, Pauly K, et al. Lifestyle medicine shared medical appointments. Am J Lifestyle Med 2021;15(1):23–7.

49. Lohnberg JA, Salcido L, Frayne S, et al. Rapid conversion to virtual obesity care in COVID-19: Impact on patient care, interdisciplinary collaboration, and training. Obes Sci Pract 2022;8(1):131–6.

50. Kuwabara A, Su S, Krauss J. Utilizing digital health technologies for patient education in lifestyle medicine. Am J Lifestyle Med 2020;14(2):137–42.

51. American College of Lifestyle Medicine. HEAL project. Lifestylemedicine.org. Available at: https://lifestylemedicine.org/project/heal-scholarship. Accessed February 12, 2023.

52. Cassoobhoy A, Sardana JJ, Benigas S, et al. Building health equity: Action steps from the American college of lifestyle medicine's health disparities solutions summit (HDSS) 2020. Am J Lifestyle Med 2022;16(1):61–75.

53. Committee on Transforming Health Care to Create Whole Health, Strategies to Assess, Scale, and Spread the Whole Person Approach to Health, Board on Health Care Services, Health and Medicine Division, National Academies of Sciences, Engineering, and Medicine, Krist AH, South-Paul J, Meisnere M. Achieving whole health: A new approach for veterans and the nation. Review 2023. https://doi.org/10.17226/26854.

Rethinking Health and Health Care
How Clinicians and Practice Groups Can Better Promote Whole Health and Well-Being for People and Communities

Alex H. Krist, MD, MPH[a,*], Jeannette E. South Paul, MD, DHL(Hon)[b],
Shawna V. Hudson, PhD[c], Marc Meisnere, MHS[d],
Sara J. Singer, PhD, MBA[e], Harold Kudler, MD[f,g]

KEYWORDS

- Health promotion • Preventive medicine • Health care delivery • Health policy
- Person-centered care • Primary health care • Practice transformation
- Integrative health

KEY POINTS

- Whole health is physical, behavioral, spiritual, and socioeconomic well-being as defined by the people served. Whole health care is an interprofessional, team-based approach anchored in trusted longitudinal relationships to promote resilience, prevent disease, and restore health that aligns with a person's life mission, aspiration, and purpose.
- Whole health systems are (1) people-centered, (2) comprehensive and holistic, (3) upstream-focused, (4) equitable and accountable, and grounded in (5) team well-being.
- Well implemented, evidence-based preventive care is a core feature of whole health care and must be integrated into all aspects of whole health systems.
- A national effort to realign conventional biomedical health care with the whole health care approach is demonstrating a range of improved outcomes.
- There are actionable ways, available now, for clinicians and practice groups to better deliver whole health to the people, families, and communities they serve.

[a] Department of Family Medicine and Population Health, Virginia Commonwealth University, Wright Regional Center for Clinical and Translational Science, Inova Health System; [b] Office of the Provost, Meharry Medical College; [c] Department of Family Medicine and Community Health, Robert Wood Johnson Medical School; [d] National Academies of Sciences, Engineering, and Medicine; [e] Department of Medicine, Stanford University School of Medicine; [f] Department of Psychiatry and Behavioral Sciences, Duke University; [g] Department of Psychiatry, Uniformed Services University of the Health Sciences
* Corresponding author. One Capitol Square, Room 631, 830 East Main Street, Richmond, VA 23219.
E-mail address: Alexander.krist@vcuhealth.org

Med Clin N Am 107 (2023) 1121–1144
https://doi.org/10.1016/j.mcna.2023.06.001
0025-7125/23/© 2023 Elsevier Inc. All rights reserved.

WHY A NEW APPROACH TO HEALTH CARE IS NEEDED

Despite spending more than other wealthy countries on health care, the United States has worse health outcomes.[1–4] US life expectancy lags behind peer nations and is declining.[5] There are stark disparities in outcomes based on race, ethnicity, and where people live, with differences of up to 18 years in life expectancy.[6,7] The high cost and poor outcomes in the United States demand change. The current biomedical focus on disease treatment with dominant fee-for-service payments does not promote well-being and disease prevention. Health care is reactive, transactional, and treats problems after they arise. New goals and a systematic reorientation of national health resources and activities are needed.

Several movements have attempted to shift the focus of health care to create better value. The World Health Organization led international efforts to redefine health around wellness, labeling it "the extent to which an individual or group is able to realize aspirations and satisfy needs to change or cope with the environment" and saying "health is a resource for everyday life, not the objective."[8,9] The patient-centered care movement advanced the idea of shifting our focus from treating diseases to addressing patient values and priorities, which has evolved to the people-centered public health approach.[10–13] Given the impact of the social determinants on health, health behaviors, and mental health, there have been many calls to better address these root causes of poor health as part of routine clinical care to prevent disease and disease progression.[14–18]

Primary care and preventive medicine, grounded in more holistic people-centered care, is the only part of the US health care system that results in longer lives and more equity.[19,20] However, even if high-quality primary care and preventive medicine is available in every community nationally, it will not fix problems with the US health care system without a larger systems approach. There are several exemplar systems-level approaches that could serve as a model for high value care across the country, such as the Department of Veterans Affairs' (VA) Whole Health System (WHS). The VA WHS changes the health care conversation from "what is the matter *with* you" to "what matters *to* you." It is a people-centered, integrative, and transformative approach intended to create and enable health and well-being by incorporating individuals' goals and priorities into their health care decisions. The care model includes peer-led support, personalized health planning, coaching, well-being courses, preventive medicine, and integrated evidence-based conventional, complementary, behavioral, and integrative practices with the goal of addressing the social determinants of health.[21–23]

Building on these movements, the National Academies of Sciences, Engineering, and Medicine (NASEM) was charged with examining the potential for improving health outcomes through a *whole health care approach* both within VA and nationally.[24] Its multidisciplinary expert committee was tasked with assessing where whole health care is being implemented, what whole health care accomplishes, and how effectively whole health approaches can be spread. This article summarizes key findings from the committee's report with a focus on actions for clinicians, practices, and practice groups to help people, families, and communities achieve whole health, with a key focus on prevention.[25]

METHODS

The 18 committee members brought diverse backgrounds, skills, and expertise including people-centered care, primary health care, preventive medicine expertise, mental and behavioral health, complementary and integrative health, health systems, veterans health, health disparities, community-based care, public health, nursing, payment policy, social work, coaching, social determinants, and health disparities.[24]

The committee held six 2-day meetings and 2 public information gathering sessions. It commissioned 3 expert papers that summarized the evidence on patient-centeredness,[26] the VA Whole Health System,[27] and lessons from other whole health implementations domestically and internationally.[28] NASEM's staff and committee members conducted a scoping literature review of more than 5000 articles to synthesize and summarize findings and conclusions. The committee's recommendations were driven by consensus followed by external peer review by 10 experts from a variety of disciplines.

WHAT IS WHOLE HEALTH AND WHOLE HEALTH CARE?

The committee's first task was to develop a definition and description of what whole health is and what is required to deliver whole health care. The committee did this by drawing from identified definitions and examples of whole health approaches.

The committee determined that...

Whole health is physical, behavioral, spiritual, and socioeconomic well-being as defined by individuals, families, and communities. To achieve this, whole health care is an interprofessional, team-based approach anchored in trusted longitudinal relationships to promote resilience, prevent disease, and restore health. It aligns with a person's life mission, aspiration, and purpose.

Having whole health is fundamentally different from being healthy in a biomedical model. Whole health is a resource for everyday life to enable people and communities to achieve their life aspirations and cope with change. Achieving whole health starts with understanding what matters to people and then builds the environment, resources, and support to help people and communities achieve their life goals.

The committee also identified 5 foundational elements needed for effective whole health care systems. These include being (1) people-centered, (2) comprehensive and holistic, (3) upstream-focused, (4) equitable and accountable, and grounded in (5) team well-being (**Table 1**). The foundational elements not only make conceptual and logical sense as essential building blocks for whole health care, but decades of robust evidence support their benefit to help people, families, and communities achieve whole health.

Evidence demonstrates that people-centered care improves the experience of receiving care, which in turn helps people to feel subjectively better and improves some physiologic measures. It also helps to create a sense of purpose and engage people as partners in their care, allowing improved self-management.[11,12,29,30] Comprehensive and holistic care is necessary to address the full spectrum of needs for diverse communities and has been shown to improve patient satisfaction, lower health care costs, reduce hospitalizations, and lower clinician and team burnout.[31,32] Addressing adverse upstream factors, such as obesity, unhealthy behaviors, sedentary lifestyle, mental health, social needs, environment, and systemic racism and sexism, is essential to prevent adverse outcomes and promote wellness. Helping people with upstream factors is complex and involves combined health, community, occupational, social services, and public health systems approaches.[14,15,17,18,33,34]

Because health inequities are a key driver of poor health, evidence shows that equity and accountability are essential for ensuring whole health. Practices and systems focused on caring for vulnerable and underserved people increase access to care and the receipt of recommended services and reduce emergency room visits and hospitalizations for those in most need.[35,36] Evidence further demonstrates that assuming

Table 1
The five foundational elements of whole health care

People-centered	Achieving a sense of purpose through longitudinal, relationship-based care People/families/communities direct goals of care Care delivered in social and cultural context of people/family/community
Comprehensive and holistic	Address all domains that affect health—acute care, chronic care, prevention, dental, vision, hearing, promoting healthy behaviors, addressing mental health, integrative medicine, social care, and spiritual care Attend to the entirety of a person/family/community's state of being Components and team members are integrated and coordinated
Upstream-focused	Multisectoral, integrated, and coordinated approach to identifying and addressing root causes of poor health Address the structures and conditions of daily life to make them more conducive to whole health
Equitable and accountable	Whole health systems need to be accountable for the health and well-being of the people, families, and communities they serve Care needs to be accessible to and high-quality for all
Team well-being	The health of the care delivery team is supported

accountability for people, family, and communities is an essential pathway to drive health systems to provide equitable care.[37] A "no wrong door" type approach, allowing people to access care through many avenues and embedding whole health supports, resources, and care where people live, work, learn, and play, further improves access and quality of care. Finally, reducing team member burnout has been shown to improve patient outcomes and quality of care.[38]

EVIDENCE SUPPORTING WHOLE HEALTH CARE SYSTEMS

The committee identified 7 US-based and 5 international-based exemplars of whole health systems that implemented and evaluated an approach consistent with the committee's definition, including the VA WHS, and had published peer-reviewed evidence demonstrating outcomes from their whole health implementation (**Table 2**). Each system operationalized the foundational elements differently based on the local environment and resources as well as the preferences and needs of the people and communities served. In all cases, the whole health system was greater than the sum of its parts, demonstrating the need for a holistic approach rather than the mere addition of multiple isolated interventions. The identified examples occurred in a range of settings spanning federally qualified health centers, health systems, government programs, and state and national programs. All programs had unique funding mechanisms beyond fee-for-service payment to allow program development such as value-based or per member per month payments, subsidies, grants, or even charitable donations (see **Table 2**). At the core of a whole health system was a clear and identified approach to strengthening primary and preventive care.

Although different studies in the published literature measured different outcomes and no single whole health approach demonstrated, or even measured, all potential benefits, the committee found evidence across the 12 approaches that whole health care had multiple benefits, including improved patient care experience and quality

Table 2
Published outcomes of implementing a whole health approach

Program	Description	Outcomes	Source of Funding
US examples of whole health care implementations			
VA Whole Health System[23,57,58,59]	See "Examples of 5 Whole Health Implementations" section	• Veterans used services and clinicians embraced approach • Improved pain and reduced opioid use for chronic pain • Improved mental health and quality of life • Greater health competence	Federal funding through congressional budgetary resources[60]
Nuka System of Care[61-63]	See "Examples of Five Whole Health Implementations" section	• More people with a primary care home • Improved access to care • Improved diabetes monitoring, immunizations, and screening • Reduced specialist use, emergency room use, and hospitalizations	Federal funding; patient services revenue (public, private, and self-pay); state of Alaska funding[64]
Kitsap Mental Health[65]	A whole health approach for people with mental illness that addresses all aspects of a person's health, including mental health, substance use, and nonpsychiatric health needs by multidisciplinary teams	• Reduced Medicare expenditures, hospitalizations, emergency room visits, and office visits per month	Contract revenue through Medicaid Managed Care; patient services revenue (public, private, and self-pay); contributions and grants[66]
Advanced Care for the Elderly (ACE) Programs[66-70]	See "Examples of Five Whole Health Implementations" section	• Reduced emergency room visits, hospitalizations, readmission rates, total bed stays in the hospital • Improved quality of life scores • Lower health care spending • Some conflicting findings across studies	Programs funded through capitated payments; Medicare Managed Care; and Medicare Shared Savings Programs (ACOs)[71-73]

(continued on next page)

Table 2
(continued)

Program	Description	Outcomes	Source of Funding
Mary's Center[74]	See "Examples of Five Whole Health Implementations" section	• Top ranked Federally Qualified Health Centers for cervical screening, child immunizations, cholesterol treatment, adolescent weight management, depression screening, and asthma treatment • 99% of teen after school programs participants graduated from high school, avoided pregnancy, attended college • Home visiting program reported "virtually no" cases of abuse or neglect after enrollment	Patient services revenue; US government grants; nonfederal grants; leased employee revenue; other contributions and grants[75]
Vermont Blueprint for Health[76,77]	Community-led whole health to improve health and well-being supported by a statutory framework, integrated systems of health care, population health, health care, care coordination, and health maintenance	• Improved adolescent well-care visits, breast and cervical cancer screening, appropriate testing for pharyngitis, diabetes eye exams, A1c testing • Reduced low value care • Reduced overall costs, driven by reduced hospital costs	Public and private insurance support[78]
National Intrepid Center of Excellence [51,79]	See "Examples of Five Whole Health Implementations" section	• Improved Neurobehavioral Symptom Inventory, post-traumatic stress disorder) Checklist, Satisfaction with Life Scale, Patient Health Questionnaire-9, Generalized Anxiety Disorder-7, Epworth Sleepiness Scale, Headache Impact Test	Federal funding[80]

International examples of whole health care implementations

Canterbury Health Pathways (New Zealand)[81,82]	Integrated whole health approach that includes resources and practitioners outside of conventional medical care, informed by communities, focused on self-management of health and a focus on helping marginalized populations	• Fewer annual hospitalizations compared to country overall • Reduced long hospital stays for people over 75 y • Reduced proportion of people over 75 y living in nursing homes • Reduced surgical wait list by improving access to care	Southern District Health Board in New Zealand[83]
South Australia Health in All Policies and South Australia Integrated Care[84,85]	Government-wide approach to consider health across sectors and policy making both inside and outside health care with a focus on upstream factors with parallel government investment in integrated care	• Increased understanding of equity and health impacts of policy among public servants • New policies passed and partially implemented to address education, employment, regional planning, healthy weight, aboriginal driving	Government of South Australia[86]
Integrated Chronic Care Model (Spain's Basque Country)[87–89]	Population health approach that used risk stratification to identify people with chronic conditions, prevention and health promotion efforts targeting chronic conditions; emphasis on self-care; integrated electronic health records (EHRs) and other methods to improve coordination and continuity; and e-visits and e-prescriptions to improve access and monitoring	• Clinicians reported system improvements (eg, care model, self-management support, clinical decision support, information systems, shared goals, patient-centered approach, etc.) • Improved quality measures • Reduced hospital use, readmission, and adverse event admission • Reduced mental health readmissions	Basque Ministry of Health[87]
Gesundes Kinzigtal Model (Germany)[90–92]	Population-based integrated care model operated via shared savings contract that includes integrated coordinated care teams, shared decision making, patient engagement through education and classes, and interdisciplinary team support	• Improved medication compliance for chronic conditions • Lower risk of osteopathic fracture • Lower risk of death • Cost savings with no decrease in quality	German health care management company and 2 statutory health insurers[93]

(continued on next page)

Table 2
(continued)

Program	Description	Outcomes	Source of Funding
EBAIS Community-Based Primary Care (Costa Rica)[94–97]	Multidisciplinary care teams assigned groups of people in different regions across the country to provide comprehensive acute, chronic, and preventive care, both at a clinic as well as in homes within the community; teams visit each household at least once a year to conduct social, demographic, and other health needs surveys, as well as to register patients in their families in a geolocated EHR	• More than 94% Costa Rican residents empaneled • Decrease in deaths from communicable disease • Reduced infant mortality • Reduced under-5 mortality • Reduced maternal mortality • Reduced adult mortality • Less health care spending than the world average • Nearly one-third of health care expenditures go to the poorest quintile of the population	Employer, employee, and government contributions; international loans and contributions[98]

measures; increased access to care, reduced emergency room use and hospitalizations; improved management of chronic pain, mental health, traumatic brain injury, and healthy aging; reduced maternal and infant mortality; improved health equity; and reduced health care expenditures (see **Table 2**).[24] The committee found more published examples of whole health approaches than expected, but systematic evaluations of how whole health care was implemented were scarce, often limited in the methods used and outcomes studied, and rarely longitudinal. Continued and more rigorous evaluations will be needed to evolve and support a nationwide effort to improve how we deliver health care.

EXAMPLES OF FIVE WHOLE HEALTH IMPLEMENTATIONS

The committee's report highlights 5 US whole health care delivery models whose program design and philosophical approach are well aligned with the committee's 5 foundational elements (**Table 3**). These examples represent a diverse spectrum of approaches, which can help to inform clinicians and practices on how they can make local whole health transformations.

Department of Veterans Affairs Whole Health System

Person centeredness is central to VA's WHS, and the entire approach centers around what matters most to each individual veteran. It is not diagnosis or disease-focused, but rather it emphasizes the whole person and prioritizes their goals and aspirations. It includes peer-led exploration of an individual's life mission, aspiration, and purpose. Needs and goals are comprehensively identified through a health inventory and health coaches coordinate and facilitate care across domains to ensure it is holistic. Resources, support, and wrap around services are provided to address upstream needs identified through the health inventory. A "Circle of Health" model guides and coordinates care; it comprises 4 parts: (1) *me*, referring to the veteran who is at the center of care, has a unique history, and is focused on what matters to them; (2) *self care*, referring to the fact that every individual has the ability to affect their own health and well-being, with WHS providing education, skills, and support for changes that are important to the veteran, (3) *professional care*, referring to the health team that assists with both prevention and treatment of disease and illness; and (4) *community*, referring to the people and groups important to the veteran and with whom they connect. The VA appears committed to ensuring that, as the WHS grows within its system, it does so with a commitment to health equity and accountability.[39] Team well-being is recognized as important with numerous individual-level interventions documented; however, the committee found that explicit efforts to address team well-being at the system level were more limited.

Nuka System of Care/Southcentral Foundation

The Nuka System of Care is an Alaska Native-owned, nonprofit federally qualified health center serving nearly 65,000 Alaska Native and American Indian people in Anchorage, Matanuska-Susitna Borough, and 55 rural villages. The Nuka system is characterized by a customer-driven whole-person care approach focused on individuals (called "customer-owners") and their families.[40] Services are woven into customers' lives and built around them, rather than around a medical office. The approach is built on comprehensive primary care, in both outpatient and home settings, as well as dentistry, outpatient behavioral health, residential behavioral health, traditional healing, complementary medicine, health education, and more. Nuka consists of a medical center—Alaska Native Medical Center's 150-bed hospital and the

Table 3
Examples of five settings that have implemented a whole health approach

Foundational Element	Components of Foundational Elements	Veterans Health Administration Whole Health System [23,39,57-59]	Nuka System of Care South Central Foundation [40-44]	Mary's Center [45-48]	National Intrepid Center of Excellence [49-51]	Advanced Care for the Elderly [52-54]
People-centered	Self-empowerment, longitudinal, relationship-based	Individualized planning	Individualized planning with "customer-owner" focus	Individualized planning to create shared expectations and goals on the outcomes	Individual skills-based education program where patients are students to be engaged in care	Individualized planning for older people to remain living independently in the community
	People family community-directed	Veterans set own health priorities	Shared responsibility for priority setting and relationship centered	Shared responsibility for priority setting, monthly community council	Shared responsibility for priority setting and relationship centered	Shared responsibility for priority setting and relationship centered
	Care delivered in social and cultural context	Peers incorporated in care team and programs provided in community	Family wellness focus, not disease centered	Hiring staff from the community to provide culturally and linguistically appropriate care	Spouses/significant others encouraged to participate in individual appointments	Focus on chronic conditions based on ongoing needs assessments to tailor care
Holistic and comprehensive	Addresses all domains that impact health	Self-administered health inventory shapes personal health plan	Access to a coordinated, comprehensive system of care	Services through community health center setting	Access to a coordinated comprehensive system of services	Access to a coordinated comprehensive system of services
	Attends to the entirety of a person, family, and community	Health coaching, skill building, self-care groups	Community centered gatherings of "Learning Circles"	Uses Social Change Model [47]	Patient story presented to care team on intake	Comprehensive care plan aligned with patient care and preferences
	Components and teams are coordinated	Allopathic, complementary and integrative health team, and peers integrated into health team	Care delivered by interprofessional teams rather than individual clinicians	Integrated behavioral health model	Allopathic and complementary and integrative health teams integrated into health team	Care delivered by interprofessional teams led by home care givers and home care workers

Upstream-focused	Identify and address root causes of poor health	Uses Circle of Health Model[22]	Social and community programs available	Social needs tracked using the Protocol for Responding to and Assessing Patients' Assets, Risks, and Experiences Tool[46]	Upstream-focused professionals included as part of interprofessional care team	Care teams monitor medical, behavioral, social, and well-being of participants
	Addresses the conditions of daily life	Resources provided to address social needs	Social needs tracked in electronic health record and resources provided for housing	Care coordination, case management, and educational programs provided	Behavioral health specialists, family counselors, social workers, and nutritionists available	Care teams meet and discuss participants whole health
Equitable and accountable	Accountable to people, families, communities	All veterans are eligible to receive Whole Health System (WHS) services	Customer-ownership model	Infrastructure for accountability and continuous quality improvement with public reporting	Care focused on individual participants	Available to individuals meeting eligibility criteria
	Accessible to all	WHS is being fully implemented system-wide	Open access scheduling, expanded hours, and electronic communication	Sliding scale feed for uninsured, catchment analysis, community needs assessment	Service members meeting criteria eligible to participate in the program	Available to seniors in some communities
Team well-being	The health of the care delivery team is supported	Well-being interventions target individual resilience	Well-being interventions available	Burnout reduction initiatives, trauma-informed practice workgroup, health equity taskforce	No published approach	No published approach

Anchorage Native Primary Care Center—and other Southcentral Foundation facilities and services. Coordinated care is delivered by interprofessional teams of primary care physicians or physician assistants, nurses, certified medical assistants, behavioral health consultants, nutritionists, HIV consultants, and appointment schedulers. Community programming support guides people through the health care system by integrating and not simply coordinating care.[41] Learning circles, community-centered gatherings based on the Alaska Native value of sharing story and listening, have been leveraged to provide more immediate access to behavioral health services and to create supportive communities.[42] There is a strong emphasis on addressing the social, environmental, and behavioral determinants of health in order to improve the overall health and well-being of customer-owners.[43] The electronic health record (EHR) tracks social needs without stigmatizing customer-owners. The system also employs universal empanelment, a hallmark of equity and accountability, as everyone in the system either self-selects or is assigned to an integrated and comprehensive care team that is accountable for their care.[44]

Mary's Center

Mary's Center is a federally qualified health center that primarily serves women and children, immigrants, low-income individuals, and uninsured or underinsured people in Washington DC and Maryland. It has a focus on ensuring personalized access, affordability, and quality in addition to understanding the person's values and wishes. Mary's Center uses the term, "participants," in recognition that people actively participate in their care and are true partners with shared expectations and goals. Design and services are determined by a patient-majority board of directors and a monthly Community Engagement Council. Staff are hired from the community to ensure culturally and linguistically appropriate care. Program participants come from roughly 50 different countries and employees come from 40 countries and speak over 35 different languages.[45] Mary's Center uses the Protocol for Responding to and Assessing Patients' Assets, Risks, and Experiences tool, which is integrated into the EHR, to collect and track the participants' social determinants of health,[46] and a Patient Care Advocate to support and coordinate access to comprehensive care. Health care, social services, family literacy programs, and educational services are holistically integrated using the "Social Change Model" to inform care, which recognizes that social and economic well-being are integral to overall wellness.[47] Care coordination and case management assist participants in obtaining food, clothing, housing, direct cash assistance, and educational programs. Mary's Center has an infrastructure for accountability and continuous quality improvement and publicly reports its clinical quality measures.[48] Burnout reduction initiatives focus on improving workflow efficiency, such as through technology adoption; building personal resilience through retreats, exercise classes, and meditation classes; and improving organizational communications through activities such as virtual town halls and intranet development. Mary's Center has a Trauma-Informed Practice Workgroup designed to create a work environment in which staff feel safe to voice concerns and address issues and convenes a Health Equity Taskforce.

National Intrepid Center of Excellence

National Intrepid Center of Excellence (NICoE) treats service members with comorbid traumatic brain injury and psychological health conditions that have not responded to previous treatment or for whom extensive treatment options are not available at their home stations. Care is delivered at the Intrepid Spirit University, which combines integrative medicine modalities with traditional care for postconcussive treatment.[49] The model views each participant as a student and clinicians as admission officers who assess each individual's needs fully, as well as the impact of the injuries on the student's family. An admissions committee comprising clinicians, neuropsychologists, behavioral health, and rehabilitation professionals develops an individualized curriculum and uses Goal Attainment Scaling collaboratively tracking students' progress.[50] The student's spouse/significant other is strongly encouraged to participate. NICoE offers comprehensive and holistic care through multiple outpatient traumatic brain injury programs. Care teams include an internist, neurologist, psychiatrist, neuropsychologist, family therapist, designated nurse specialist, audiologist, art therapist, chaplain, licensed clinical social worker, nutrition specialist, occupational therapist, optometrist, physical therapist, recreational therapist, sleep medicine physician, and speech and language pathologists.[51] NICoE provides conventional medical and alternative treatments such as group counseling, psychoeducation, yoga, Tai Chi, and a canine program. NICoE's interprofessional care team includes behavioral health specialists and family counselors, and may include a licensed clinical social worker, nutritionist, and sleep medicine physician.

Advanced Care for the Elderly

Advanced Care for the Elderly is a series of programs for older adults to help people meet their health care needs in the community instead of going to a nursing home and includes the Program of All-Inclusive Care for the Elderly , the Geriatric Resources for Assessment and Care of Elders program, and the House Calls program. Interdisciplinary care team members include a primary care clinician, nurse, social worker, physical therapist, occupational therapist, recreational therapist or activity coordinator, dietitian, center supervisor, nursing aids, and drivers. Team members meet regularly to exchange information and review and update patient's plan as their needs change.[52] Frequent contact allows close monitoring of chronic conditions, ongoing needs assessment, adaptation of care plans, and an opportunity for care team members to build close, longitudinal relationships with program participants.[53] Homecare workers are included as part of the team and can help with light housekeeping, personal care, light meals preparation, feeding, medication reminders, laundry, and escort assistance to medical appointments. Care plans address a standard set of biopsychosocial, functional, and other issues relevant to the health of frail older adults. Numerous upstream factors impact the elderly and are routinely incorporated as part of the care plan.[54]

CHANGES CLINICIANS AND PRACTICES CAN MAKE TO MOVE TOWARD A WHOLE HEALTH APPROACH

The committee made multiple recommendations to create a national, state, and local roadmap on how to scale and spread a whole health care approach (**Table 4**). These are fully detailed in the report.[25] Each recommendation has an identified actor to carry out the recommendation and defined outcomes to demonstrate success for the recommendation. For busy clinicians and practice groups, these recommendations and goals may seem out of reach, aspirational, and beyond control. However, there are concrete actions that clinicians and practices can take now to implement a whole health care approach locally that will help the people, families, and communities they serve to better achieve whole health. Clinicians and practices starting this process can serve as a grass roots catalyst to create whole health approaches in their community.

Table 4
Actions clinicians and practice groups can take now to implement a whole health care approach

Committee Recommendation	National Actions	Clinician and Practice Actions
COMMIT to the *shared purpose* of helping people achieve whole health	Federal agencies addressing health and social services, state and local governments, health systems, social services, community programs, and external environment actors (payers, corporations, educators, and others) should make whole health a core value	• Name your care delivery approach a "whole health approach" • Make whole health part of your core mission statement • Create a vision and roadmap for delivering whole health • Gain leadership and staff buy-in • Identifying champions to lead needed transformations • Instill whole health in day-to-day culture
PREPARE for a *whole health* approach to care	Health care systems, community programs, social services, and public health organizations committed to helping people achieve whole health should ensure that all sites are ready to offer whole health care to the people, families, and communities they serve	• Assess your organization and team members' readiness • Identify the elements of current care that will need to change to transition from conventional to whole health care • Determine available resources in your practice and community • Establish your interprofessional teams • Include the people and communities you serve in your whole health care design
INTEGRATE *across systems, services, and time* to support whole health care throughout the lifespan	Health care systems should create and strengthen the infrastructure needed to partner with community programs, social care, and public health systems	• Create care partnerships between the clinical, social services, and community programs in your community • Develop the workflow and processes to collaborate, share information, and coordinate resources • Develop structural elements that support integration like patient and family advisory councils, health coaches, peer-support specialists, and health information technology

DELIVER *all foundational elements* of whole health care	• Health care systems, community programs, social services, and public health organizations should model and advance whole health approaches after the other early adopters • Building on its existing health center program, the Health Resources and Services Administration should lead the scale and spread of whole health care in the community	• Implement high-quality primary care model[19] • Create people-centered care through longitudinal relationships • Design tailored care plans with patients • Co-locate clinical and mental health care • Assess social needs and partner with community programs to deliver social services • Develop substance use interventions • Provide accessible rehabilitative services • Integrate complementary and integrative health services • Ensure efficient hand-off procedures between care settings
EVALUATE to iteratively refine whole health care systems and *create generalizable knowledge*	• Systems fielding whole health should systematically and continuously evaluate and participate in external evaluations of their implementation and adaptations • The Agency for Healthcare Research and Quality should fund research to evaluate whole health care as well as research that disseminates evidence on whole health practices	• Identify measures of success and accountability • Prospectively, consider comparison groups (pre–post, staged implementation, control practices/clinicians) • Collect data to longitudinally track outcomes • Collect data to track how the whole health approach is implemented and adapted and the impact on outcomes • Look for national or regional evaluation programs to participate in
DESIGN public and private sector *policies and payment* to support whole health as a common good and whole health care as a way of achieving whole health	The Department of Veterans Affairs, in partnership with the Department of Health and Human Services, should create a national Center for Whole Health Innovation to design and advance the policies and payments for whole health care	• Participate in experiments and demonstration projects to create whole health • Use personal whole health implementation experience to inform local community's/system's whole health approach • Use personal whole health implementation experience to inform Center of Whole Health Innovation efforts

The national recommendations to scale and spread whole health care are framed around 6 goals, many of which can be directly implemented by clinicians and practices. They include:

1. COMMIT to the *shared purpose* of helping people achieve whole health. Engagement, support, buy-in, and prioritization from the bottom up and top down are needed to enable the cultural and structural transformations necessary to scale and spread a system of whole health care.
2. PREPARE for a *whole health* approach to care. Interprofessional teams, organizations, and systems need to understand where they are developmentally on the trajectory to delivering whole health care and what they need to change to deliver whole health care.
3. INTEGRATE *across systems, services, and time* to support whole health care throughout the lifespan. Achieving whole health will require support in all settings throughout peoples' lifespan, and within and across the communities to ensure holistic and comprehensive care.
4. DELIVER *all foundational elements* of whole health care. Each foundational element of whole health care is essential and interdependent, and successful whole health systems need to attend to all 5 elements.
5. EVALUATE to iteratively refine whole health care systems and *create generalizable knowledge*. The understanding of how to best deliver whole health care is evolving rapidly; so evaluating, adapting approaches efficiently, and sharing learnings will be essential for national success.
6. "DESIGN public and private sector *policies and payment* to support whole health as a common good and whole health care as a way of achieving whole health." Scaling and spreading whole health care throughout the United States will not be possible without realigning infrastructure, policies, and payment to support, promote, and fund the provision of the foundational elements of whole health care.

Committing (goal 1) to a shared purpose starts with understanding what whole health is and then acting to demonstrate a commitment to a whole health approach. Simple actions like naming how care is delivered to a whole health approach or including whole health as part of a core mission statement can begin a cultural shift from a biomedical to whole health mindset (see **Table 4**). *Preparing* (goal 2) includes assessing the current state of care delivery; identifying gaps that need to be addressed to adopt a whole health approach; allying with services and resources already available in the local conventional health system social services agencies, and community programs; and assembling a whole health interprofessional team. The interprofessional care team is an essential structure to support whole health and includes clinicians and nonclinicians who collaborate across disciplines and settings.[55] Team composition will depend on the needs of local people and communities and would likely benefit from being organized around a core team, an extended health care team, and an extended community care team.[56] Core team could include the person seeking whole health, that person's family and informal caregivers, and the team members most directly involved in helping the individual achieve their whole health goals and addressing the person's most pressing health needs. Extended whole health care teams include members and services more peripheral to an individual's care plan but still involved on an as-needed basis to augment the core team. Community care team members could include community health workers; social support professionals to help with housing, food insecurity, childcare, elder care, educational, training, and employment needs; peer-support specialists; home health aides; disability support professionals; and religious or spiritual supports, among others.

By definition, a whole health approach will require collaboration across clinical care, social services, and community programs, which involves *integration* (goal 3) of services to create a comprehensive and holistic experience. Clinicians and practices can develop a variety of structural elements needed to support integration including patient and family advisory councils, health coaches, peer-support specialists, and EHR and health information technology support (see **Table 4**). To *deliver* (goal 4) all the foundational elements of whole health care, clinicians and practices can model their approaches after what others have done (see **Tables 2** and **3**). The National Academies' report identified multiple specific changes that practices could make to move toward a whole health approach such as ensuring primary care is following the high-quality primary care model,[19] creating people-centered care through longitudinal relationships and designing with patients tailored care plans, co-locating clinical and mental health care, routinely assessing social needs and partnering with community programs to deliver social services, developing substance use interventions, providing accessible rehabilitative services, integrating complementary and integrative health services, and ensuring efficient hand-off procedures between care settings.

There is much to learn about how to best deliver whole health care and what funding models will be needed to support it. It will be critical for practices and health systems implementing whole health to *evaluate* (goal 5) both the outcomes and the process for transforming their care delivery approach. Participating in regional or national evaluations is one pathway to do this. Clinicians and practices can also do their own evaluation. Key steps will be to prospectively identify measures of success, include valid comparison groups, and longitudinally collect data to determine not only what works and what does not work but also the mechanisms underlying change in outcomes. These types of evaluations will be essential to *design* (goal 6) the policies and payment for whole health. Additionally, having piloted and locally implemented whole health approaches, clinicians and practices can serve as local leaders in informing their community's/system's whole health approach.

SUMMARY

Whole health is a common good that benefits people, families, and communities. Essential to whole health is a transition from reactive disease-focused care to proactive preventive care to promote wellness. Scaling and spreading whole health care to ensure everyone can access needed services is a tall task and will take seismic cultural, structural, and process transformations. These include how to think about what it means to be healthy, how to deliver health, who is accountable for delivering health, and how to measure success. Multisector collaboration and investment on national and local levels are needed, and clinicians and practices can make changes now to better align their care with a whole health approach.

CLINICS CARE POINTS

- Adopt Whole Health as part of your practice's mission and approach to care.
- Model your Whole Health approach to care after existing early adopters of Whole Health care.
- Prospectively plan to measure the implementation and outcomes of your Whole Health approach to better inform your design and help others learn about best approaches.

CONSENT FOR PUBLICATION

Consent provided by authors; not required by funders or National Academies of Sciences, Engineering, and Medicine.

AVAILABILITY OF DATA AND MATERIAL

Not applicable at this time as no primary data are collected.

CONFLICT OF INTEREST

None.

ADDITIONAL CONTRIBUTIONS

This article reflects the opinion of the full NASEM's committee members, who participated in developing the report, *Achieving Whole Health: A New Approach for Veterans and the Nation*. Committee members include Alex Krist, Jeanette South-Paul, Andrew Bazemore, Tammy Chang, Margaret Chesney, Deborah Cohen, Seiji Hayashi, Felicia Hill-Briggs, Shawna Hudson, Carlos Roberto Jaen, Christopher Koller, Harold Kudler, Sandy Leake, Patricia Lillis, Ajus Ninan, Pamela Schweitzer, Sara Singer, and Zirui Song. Additionally, we would like to thank the National Academies' staff and fellow (Marjani Cephus, Tochi Ogbu-Mbadiugha, Arzoo Tayyeb, Sharyl Nass, and Alexander Melamed), authors of commissioned papers (Asaf Bitton, Denise Hynes, and Moira Stewart), and science writer (Joseph Alper). The views expressed within this article do not necessarily represent the views of the NASEM, the National Research Council, or any of their constituent units.

The National Academies study was funded by the Department of Veterans Affairs, Samueli Foundation, and Whole Health Institute.

FUNDING/SUPPORT
Role of the Funder/Sponsor

The study sponsors for the National Academy of Sciences, Engineering, and Medicine Whole Health report included the U.S. Department of Veterans Affairs, Samueli Foundation, and Whole Health Institute.

REFERENCES

1. Institute of Medicine and National Research Council. U.S. Health in International Perspective: Shorter Lives, Poorer Health. Washington, DC: The National Academies Press; 2013. https://doi.org/10.17226/13497.
2. McGlynn EA, Asch SM, Adams J, et al. The quality of health care delivered to adults in the United States. N Engl J Med 2003;348(26):2635–45.
3. Schuster MA, McGlynn EA, Brook RH. How good is the quality of health care in the United States? 1998. Milbank Q 2005;83(4):843–95.
4. Herbstman BJ, Pincus HA. Measuring mental healthcare quality in the United States: a review of initiatives. Curr Opin Psychiatry 2009;22(6):623–30.
5. Woolf SH, Schoomaker H. Life Expectancy and Mortality Rates in the United States, 1959-2017. JAMA 2019;322(20):1996–2016.
6. Collaborators GUHD. Life expectancy by county, race, and ethnicity in the USA, 2000-19: a systematic analysis of health disparities. Lancet 2022;400(10345): 25–38.

7. de Mestral C. Considerations for County-Level Inequalities in Life Expectancy. JAMA Intern Med 2017;177(11):1697–8.

8. World Health Organization. Health promotion : a discussion document on the concept and principles : summary report of the Working Group on Concept and Principles of Health Promotion, Copenhagen, 9-13 July 1984. 1984. January 2022. Available at: https://apps.who.int/iris/handle/10665/107835

9. World Health Organization. Basic Documents. 49th edition. Geneva, Switzerland: World Health Organization; 2020.

10. Stewart M, Brown JB, Weston WW, et al. Patient-centered medicine: transforming the clinical method. Thousand Oaks, CA: Sage Publications, Inc.; 1995.

11. Stewart M. Patient-centered medicine: transforming the clinical method. Third edition. London: Radcliffe Publishing; 2014. p. 426.

12. Stewart M, Brown JB, Donner A, et al. The impact of patient-centered care on outcomes. J Fam Pract 2000;49(9):796–804.

13. World Health Organization. Framework on integrated, people-centred health services. Geneva, Switzerland: World Health Organization; 2016.

14. Landon BE, Grumbach K, Wallace PJ. Integrating public health and primary care systems: potential strategies from an IOM report. JAMA 2012;308(5):461–2.

15. National Academies of Sciences, Engineering, and Medicine. 2016. A Framework for Educating Health Professionals to Address the Social Determinants of Health. Washington, DC: The National Academies Press. https://doi.org/10.17226/21923.

16. WHO Commission on Social Determinants of Health., World Health Organization. Closing the gap in a generation : health equity through action on the social determinants of health : Commission on Social Determinants of Health final report, 246. World Health Organization, Commission on Social Determinants of Health; 2008. https://www.who.int/publications/i/item/WHO-IER-CSDH-08.1.

17. Davidson KW, Kemper AR, Doubeni CA, et al. Developing Primary Care-Based Recommendations for Social Determinants of Health: Methods of the U.S. Preventive Services Task Force. Ann Intern Med 2020;173(6):461–7.

18. Krist AH, Davidson KW, Ngo-Metzger Q, et al. Social Determinants as a Preventive Service: U.S. Preventive Services Task Force Methods Considerations for Research. Am J Prev Med 2019;57(6 Suppl 1):S6–12.

19. National Academies of Sciences Engineering and Medicine. Implementing High-Quality Primary Care: Rebuilding the Foundation of Health Care. National Academies Press. Accessed May, 2021. https://www.nationalacademies.org/our-work/implementing-high-quality-primary-care

20. Phillips RL Jr, McCauley LA, Koller CF. Implementing High-Quality Primary Care: A Report From the National Academies of Sciences, Engineering, and Medicine. JAMA 2021. https://doi.org/10.1001/jama.2021.7430.

21. Gaudet T, Kligler B. Whole Health in the Whole System of the Veterans Administration: How Will We Know We Have Reached This Future State? J Altern Complement Med 2019;25(S1):S7–11.

22. Jonas WB, Rosenbaum E. The Case for Whole-Person Integrative Care. Medicina (Kaunas). 2021;57(7). https://doi.org/10.3390/medicina57070677.

23. Bokhour BG, Hyde J, Kligler B, et al. From patient outcomes to system change: Evaluating the impact of VHA's implementation of the Whole Health System of Care. Health Serv Res 2022;57(Suppl 1):53–65.

24. Transforming Health Care to Create Whole Health: Strategies to Assess, Scale, and Spread the Whole Person Approach to Health. National Academy of Science, Engineering, and Medicine. Accessed Feb, 2023. https://www.natlonalacademies.org/

our-work/transforming-health-care-to-create-whole-health-strategies-to-assess-scale-and-spread-the-whole-person-approach-to-health

25. National Academies of Sciences Engineering and Medicine. Achieving whole health: a new approach for veterans and the nation. Washington, DC: National Academies Press; 2023.

26. Stewart M. Evidence on patient-centeredness, patient-centered systems, and implementation and scaling of whole person health. National Academies of Science, Engineering, and Medicine. Accessed Mar, 2023. https://nap.nationalacademies.org/resource/26854/Stewart_NASEM_Commissioned_Paper.pdf

27. Hynes DM. Whole health in VA Health Care: Insights on implementation, research, and future evaluations. National Academies of Science, Engineering, and Medicine. Accessed Mar, 2023. https://nap.nationalacademies.org/resource/26854/Hynes_Commissioned_Paper.pdf

28. Bitton A. Lessons from other health systems for whole health. National Academies of Science, Engineering, and Medicine. Accessed Mar, 2023. https://nap.nationalacademies.org/resource/26854/Bitton_NASEM_Commissioned_Paper.pdf

29. Smith SM, Wallace E, Clyne B, et al. Interventions for improving outcomes in patients with multimorbidity in primary care and community setting: a systematic review. Syst Rev 2021;10(1):271.

30. McMillan SS, Kendall E, Sav A, et al. Patient-centered approaches to health care: a systematic review of randomized controlled trials. Med Care Res Rev 2013; 70(6):567–96.

31. Starfield B, Shi L, Macinko J. Contribution of primary care to health systems and health. Milbank Q 2005;83(3):457–502.

32. Bazemore A, Petterson S, Peterson LE, et al. More Comprehensive Care Among Family Physicians is Associated with Lower Costs and Fewer Hospitalizations. Ann Fam Med 2015;13(3):206–13.

33. Marmot M, Friel S, Bell R, et al. Closing the gap in a generation: health equity through action on the social determinants of health. Lancet 2008;372(9650): 1661–9.

34. Krist AH, Davidson KW, Ngo-Metzger Q. What evidence do we need before recommending routine screening for social determinants of health? Am Fam Physician 2019;99(10):602–5.

35. Falik M, Needleman J, Wells BL, et al. Ambulatory care sensitive hospitalizations and emergency visits: experiences of Medicaid patients using federally qualified health centers. Med Care 2001;39(6):551–61.

36. Richard P, Shin P, Beeson T, et al. Quality and Cost of Diabetes Mellitus Care in Community Health Centers in the United States. PLoS One 2015;10(12): e0144075.

37. Crook H, Whitaker R, Bleser W, et al. The Past Decade of Paying for Value : From the Affordable Care Act to COVID-19. N C Med J 2020;81(6):381–5.

38. National Academies of Sciences Engineering and Medicine. Taking Action Against Clinician Burnout: A Systems Approach to Professional Well-Being. Washington DC: The National Academies Press; 2019.

39. Kligler B, Hyde J, Gantt C, et al. The Whole Health Transformation at the Veterans Health Administration: Moving From "What's the Matter With You?" to "What Matters to You? Med Care 2022;60(5):387–91.

40. Gottlieb K. The Nuka System of Care: improving health through ownership and relationships. Int J Circumpolar Health 2013;72(1):21118.

41. Eby DK. Primary Care at the Alaska Native Medical Center: A Fully Deployed "New Model" of Primary Care. International journal of circumpolar health 2007; 66(18154227):4–13.
42. Southcentral Foundation. Learning Circles: A Tool for Support and Personal Growth, 2022. Available at: https://scfnuka.com/learning-circles-a-tool-for-support-and-personal-growth/
43. Southcentral Foundation Nuka System of Care. Addressing the Impact of Social Determinants of Health. 2022. Available at: https://scfnuka.com/addressing-the-impact-of-social-determinants-of-health/
44. Driscoll DL, Hiratsuka V, Johnston JM, et al. Process and Outcomes of Patient-Centered Medical Care With Alaska Native People at Southcentral Foundation. Ann Fam Med 2013;11(Suppl_1):S41–9.
45. Mary's Center for Maternal and Childcare, Inc. MC2 Community Development Corporation. Audit report: for the year ended December 31, 2021. Available at: https://projects.propublica.org/nonprofits/display_audit/7592120211. Accessed April, 2023.
46. PRAPARE. PRAPARE Overview. 2022, 2022. https://prapare.org/. Accessed May 13, 2022.
47. Galvez M, Leopold J, Okeke C, Oneto A. Three Decades of Mary's Center's Social Change Model. 2019:1-60. September 16, 2019. https://www.urban.org/sites/default/files/publication/101041/three_decades_of_marys_centers_social_change_model_3.pdf
48. HRSA. 2020. Health Center Program Uniform Data System (UDS) data overview. Available at: https://data.hrsa.gov/tools/data-reporting/program data. Accessed July 14, 2023.
49. Lee KM, Greenhalgh WM, Sargent P, et al. Unique Features of the US Department of Defense Multidisciplinary Concussion Clinics. J Head Trauma Rehabil 2019;34(6).
50. Turner-Stokes L. Goal attainment scaling (GAS) in rehabilitation: a practical guide. Clin Rehabil 2009;23(4):362–70.
51. DeGraba TJ, Williams K, Koffman R, et al. Efficacy of an Interdisciplinary Intensive Outpatient Program in Treating Combat-Related Traumatic Brain Injury and Psychological Health Conditions. Front Neurol 2020;11:580182.
52. On Lok. About On Lok PACE: Providing Senior Care. 2022. Updated September 24, 2020 https://onlok.org/pace/about-on-lok-pace/. Accessed April 20, 2022, 2022.
53. Gross DL, Temkin-Greener H, Kunitz S, et al. The growing pains of integrated health care for the elderly: lessons from the expansion of PACE. Milbank Q 2004;82(2):257–82.
54. Boult C, Wieland GD. Comprehensive Primary Care for Older Patients With Multiple Chronic Conditions. JAMA 2010;304(17):1936.
55. Gittell JH, Beswick J, Goldmann D, et al. Teamwork methods for accountable care: relational coordination and TeamSTEPPS(R). Health Care Manage Rev 2015;40(2):116–25.
56. Kerrissey M, Novikov Z, Tietschert MV, et al. When perceived team boundaries blur: Inconsistent perceptions and implications for performance. Acad Manag Proc 2022;1:17982.
57. Purcell N, Zamora K, Bertenthal D, et al. How VA Whole Health Coaching Can Impact Veterans' Health and Quality of Life: A Mixed-Methods Pilot Program Evaluation. Glob Adv Health Med 2021;10. https://doi.org/10.1177/2164956121998283. 2164956121998283.

58. Parisi A, Roberts RL, Hanley AW, et al. Mindfulness-Oriented Recovery Enhancement for Addictive Behavior, Psychiatric Distress, and Chronic Pain: A Multilevel Meta-Analysis of Randomized Controlled Trials. Mindfulness (N Y). 2022;13(10): 2396–412.

59. Garland EL, Hanley AW, Nakamura Y, et al. Mindfulness-Oriented Recovery Enhancement vs Supportive Group Therapy for Co-occurring Opioid Misuse and Chronic Pain in Primary Care: A Randomized Clinical Trial. JAMA Intern Med 2022;182(4):407–17.

60. USAspending.gov. U.S. Department of Veterans Affairs. Accessed Apr, 2023. https://www.usaspending.gov/agency/department-of-veterans-affairs?fy=2023

61. Driscoll DL, Hiratsuka V, Johnston JM, et al. Process and outcomes of patient-centered medical care with Alaska Native people at Southcentral Foundation. Ann Fam Med 2013;11(Suppl 1):S41–9.

62. Johnston JM, Smith JJ, Hiratsuka VY, et al. Tribal implementation of a patient-centred medical home model in Alaska accompanied by decreased hospital use. Int J Circumpolar Health 2013;72. https://doi.org/10.3402/ijch.v72i0.20960.

63. SCF (Southcentral Foundation). The impact of relationship-based care. Accessed Mar, 2023. https://scfnuka.com/impact-relationship-based-care/

64. Southcentral Foundation. Consolidated financial statements, supplemental information, and compliance reports: years ended September 30, 2021 and 2020 https://projects.propublica.org/nonprofits/display_audit/11597120211. Accessed Apr, 2023.

65. Bouchery EE, Siegwarth AW, Natzke B, et al. Implementing a Whole Health Model in a Community Mental Health Center: Impact on Service Utilization and Expenditures. Psychiatr Serv 2018;69(10):1075–80.

66. Services KMH. Audit of consolidated financial statements: Years ended June 30, 2022 and 2021 https://projects.propublica.org/nonprofits/display_audit/22949820221. Accessed Apr, 2023.

67. Counsell SR, Callahan CM, Clark DO, et al. Geriatric care management for low-income seniors: a randomized controlled trial. JAMA 2007;298(22):2623–33.

68. Counsell SR, Callahan CM, Tu W, et al. Cost analysis of the Geriatric Resources for Assessment and Care of Elders care management intervention. J Am Geriatr Soc 2009;57(8):1420–6.

69. Melnick GA, Green L, Rich J. House Calls: California Program For Homebound Patients Reduces Monthly Spending, Delivers Meaningful Care. Health Aff 2016;35(1):28–35.

70. Arku D, Felix M, Warholak T, et al. Program of All-Inclusive Care for the Elderly (PACE) versus Other Programs: A Scoping Review of Health Outcomes. Geriatrics 2022;7(2). https://doi.org/10.3390/geriatrics7020031.

71. Bielaszka-DuVernay C. The 'GRACE' model: in-home assessments lead to better care for dual eligibles. Health Aff 2011;30(3):431–4.

72. Cornwell T. House Calls Are Reaching the Tipping Point - Now We Need the Workforce. J Patient Cent Res Rev. Summer 2019;6(3):188–91.

73. Centers for Medicare and Medicaid Services. PACE. https://www.cms.gov/outreach-and-education/american-indian-alaska-native/aian/ltss-ta-center/info/pace. Accessed Apr, 2023

74. Galvez M, Leopold J, Okeke C, Oneto A, Aron LY, López R. Three decades of Mary's Center's social change model https://www.urban.org/research/publication/three-decades-marys-centers-social-change-model. Accessed Mar, 2023.

75. Mary's Center for Maternal and Childcare, Inc. MC2 Community Development Corporation. Audit report: for the year ended December 31, 2021. https://projects.propublica.org/nonprofits/display_audit/7592120211. Accessed Apr, 2023

76. Jones C, Finison K, McGraves-Lloyd K, et al. Vermont's Community-Oriented All-Payer Medical Home Model Reduces Expenditures and Utilization While Delivering High-Quality Care. Popul Health Manag 2016;19(3):196–205.

77. Vermont Blueprint for Heath. About the Blueprint for Health. https://blueprintforhealth.vermont.gov/about-blueprint. Accessed Mar, 2023

78. *Report to the Vermont Legislature: Annual report on Blueprint for health*. https://legislature.vermont.gov/assets/Legislative-Reports/2022-Blueprint-for-Health-Annual-Report.pdf.

79. Ayer L, Farris C, Farmer CM, et al. Care Transitions to and from the National Intrepid Center of Excellence (NICoE) for Service Members with Traumatic Brain Injury. Rand Health Q 2015;5(2):12.

80. Defense Health Program. Operation and Maintenance. Defense-Wide Fiscal Year (FY) 2023 President's Budget Introductory. Statement 2023;. https://comptroller.defense.gov/Portals/45/Documents/defbudget/fy2023/budget_justification/pdfs/09_Defense_Health_Program/00-DHP_Vols_I_II_and_IV_PB23.pdf.

81. McGeoch G, Shand B, Gullery C, et al. Hospital avoidance: an integrated community system to reduce acute hospital demand. Prim Health Care Res Dev 2019;20:e144.

82. Gullery C, Hamilton G. Towards integrated person-centred healthcare - the Canterbury journey. Future Hosp J 2015;2(2):111–6.

83. Stokes T, Tumilty E, Doolan-Noble F, et al. HealthPathways Implementation in a New Zealand health region: a qualitative study using the Consolidated Framework for Implementation Research. BMJ Open 2018;8(12):e025094.

84. Baum F, Delany-Crowe T, MacDougall C, et al. To what extent can the activities of the South Australian Health in All Policies initiative be linked to population health outcomes using a program theory-based evaluation? BMC Publ Health 2019;19(1):88.

85. van Eyk H, Harris E, Baum F, et al. In All Policies in South Australia-Did It Promote and Enact an Equity Perspective? Int J Environ Res Public Health 2017;14(11). https://doi.org/10.3390/ijerph14111288.

86. Government of South Australia. Wellbeing SA 2021-2022 annual report. September 29, 2022. Accessed Apr, 2023. https://www.wellbeingsa.sa.gov.au/about-wellbeing-sa/governance-reporting

87. Polanco NT, Zabalegui IB, Irazusta IP, et al. Building integrated care systems: a case study of Bidasoa Integrated Health Organisation. Int J Integr Care 2015;15:e026.

88. Mateo-Abad M, Gonzalez N, Fullaondo A, et al. Impact of the CareWell integrated care model for older patients with multimorbidity: a quasi-experimental controlled study in the Basque Country. BMC Health Serv Res 2020;20(1):613.

89. Izagirre-Olaizola J, Hernando-Saratxaga G, Aguirre-Garcia MS. Integration of health care in the Basque Country during COVID-19: the importance of an integrated care management approach in times of emergency. Prim Health Care Res Dev 2021;22:e39.

90. Marill MC. From Rural Germany, Integrated Care Grows Into A Global Model. Health Aff 2020;39(8):1282–8.

91. Schubert I, Siegel A, Koster I, et al. [Evaluation of the population-based 'Integrated Health Care System Gesundes Kinzigtal' (IHGK). Findings on health care quality based on administrative data]. Z Evid Fortbild Qual Gesundhwes 2016;117:27–37. https://doi.org/10.1016/j.zefq.2016.06.003. Evaluation der

populationsbezogenen 'Integrierten Versorgung Gesundes Kinzigtal' (IVGK). Ergebnisse zur Versorgungsqualitat auf der Basis von Routinedaten.

92. Schubert I, Stelzer D, Siegel A, et al. Ten-Year Evaluation of the Population-Based Integrated Health Care System Gesundes Kinzigtal. Dtsch Arztebl Int 2021; 118(27–28):465–72.

93. Hildebrandt H, Hermann C, Knittel R, et al. Gesundes Kinzigtal integrated care: Improving population health by a shared health gain approach and a shared savings contract. Int J Integrated Care 2010;10:e046.

94. VanderZanden A, Pesec M, Abrams M, et al. What does community-oriented primary health care look like? Lessons from Costa Rica. Commonwealth Fund https://www.commonwealthfund.org/publications/case-study/2021/mar/community-oriented-primary-care-lessons-costa-rica. Accessed Mar, 2023.

95. Pesec M, Ratcliffe HL, Karlage A, et al. Primary Health Care That Works: The Costa Rican Experience. Health Aff 2017;36(3):531–8.

96. Spigel L, Pesec M, Villegas Del Carpio O, et al. Implementing sustainable primary healthcare reforms: strategies from Costa Rica. BMJ Glob Health 2020;5(8). https://doi.org/10.1136/bmjgh-2020-002674.

97. Unger JP, De Paepe P, Buitron R, et al. Costa Rica: achievements of a heterodox health policy. Am J Public Health 2008;98(4):636–43.

98. Cuccia L, Chadwick J, Hassan A, Kim A, Sivarajan R, Wong V. Costa Rica's Health Care Reform: Impact and Success of the EBAIS Model https://mghjournal.com/2020/09/19/vol-viii-costa-ricas-health-care-reform-impact-and-success-of-the-ebais-model/. Accessed Apr, 2023.

UNITED STATES POSTAL SERVICE® Statement of Ownership, Management, and Circulation (All Periodicals Publications Except Requester Publications)

1. Publication Title	2. Publication Number		3. Filing Date
MEDICAL CLINICS IN NORTH AMERICA	337 — 340		9/13/2023

4. Issue Frequency	5. Number of Issues Published Annually	6. Annual Subscription Price
JAN, MAR, MAY, JUL, SEP, NOV	6	$332.00

7. Complete Mailing Address of Known Office of Publication (Not printer) (Street, city, county, state, and ZIP+4®)

ELSEVIER INC.
230 Park Avenue, Suite 800
New York, NY 10169

Contact Person
Malathi Samayan
Telephone (Include area code)
+91 42594507

8. Complete Mailing Address of Headquarters or General Business Office of Publisher (Not printer)

ELSEVIER INC.
230 Park Avenue, Suite 800
New York, NY 10169

9. Full Names and Complete Mailing Addresses of Publisher, Editor, and Managing Editor (Do not leave blank)

Publisher (Name and complete mailing address)
Dolores Meloni, ELSEVIER INC.
1600 JOHN F KENNEDY BLVD. SUITE 1600
PHILADELPHIA, PA 19103-2899

Editor (Name and complete mailing address)
TAYLOR HAYES, ELSEVIER INC.
1600 JOHN F KENNEDY BLVD. SUITE 1600
PHILADELPHIA, PA 19103-2899

Managing Editor (Name and complete mailing address)
PATRICK MANLEY, ELSEVIER INC.
1600 JOHN F KENNEDY BLVD. SUITE 1600
PHILADELPHIA, PA 19103-2899

10. Owner (Do not leave blank. If the publication is owned by a corporation, give the name and address of the corporation immediately followed by the names and addresses of all stockholders owning or holding 1 percent or more of the total amount of stock. If not owned by a corporation, give the names and addresses of the individual owners. If owned by a partnership or other unincorporated firm, give its name and address as well as those of each individual owner. If the publication is published by a nonprofit organization, give its name and address.)

Full Name	Complete Mailing Address
WHOLLY OWNED SUBSIDIARY OF REED/ELSEVIER, US HOLDINGS	1600 JOHN F KENNEDY BLVD. SUITE 1600 PHILADELPHIA, PA 19103-2899

11. Known Bondholders, Mortgagees, and Other Security Holders Owning or Holding 1 Percent or More of Total Amount of Bonds, Mortgages, or Other Securities. If none, check box. ▶ ☐ None

Full Name	Complete Mailing Address
N/A	

12. Tax Status (For completion by nonprofit organizations authorized to mail at nonprofit rates) (Check one)
The purpose, function, and nonprofit status of this organization and the exempt status for federal income tax purposes:
☒ Has Not Changed During Preceding 12 Months
☐ Has Changed During Preceding 12 Months (Publisher must submit explanation of change with this statement)

PS Form 3526, July 2014 (Page 1 of 4 (see instructions page 4)) PSN: 7530-01-000-9931   PRIVACY NOTICE: See our privacy policy on www.usps.com.

13. Publication Title			14. Issue Date for Circulation Data Below
MEDICAL CLINICS IN NORTH AMERICA			JULY 2023

15. Extent and Nature of Circulation			Average No. Copies Each Issue During Preceding 12 Months	No. Copies of Single Issue Published Nearest to Filing Date
a. Total Number of Copies (Net press run)			273	249
b. Paid Circulation (By Mail and Outside the Mail)	(1)	Mailed Outside-County Paid Subscriptions Stated on PS Form 3541 (Include paid distribution above nominal rate, advertiser's proof copies, and exchange copies)	181	161
	(2)	Mailed In-County Paid Subscriptions Stated on PS Form 3541 (Include paid distribution above nominal rate, advertiser's proof copies, and exchange copies)	0	0
	(3)	Paid Distribution Outside the Mails Including Sales Through Dealers and Carriers, Street Vendors, Counter Sales, and Other Paid Distribution Outside USPS®	68	57
	(4)	Paid Distribution by Other Classes of Mail Through the USPS (e.g., First-Class Mail®)	14	21
c. Total Paid Distribution [Sum of 15b (1), (2), (3), and (4)]		▶	263	239
d. Free or Nominal Rate Distribution (By Mail and Outside the Mail)	(1)	Free or Nominal Rate Outside-County Copies included on PS Form 3541	9	9
	(2)	Free or Nominal Rate In-County Copies Included on PS Form 3541	0	0
	(3)	Free or Nominal Rate Copies Mailed at Other Classes Through the USPS (e.g., First-Class Mail)	0	0
	(4)	Free or Nominal Rate Distribution Outside the Mail (Carriers or other means)	1	1
e. Total Free or Nominal Rate Distribution (Sum of 15d (1), (2), (3) and (4))		▶	10	10
f. Total Distribution (Sum of 15c and 15e)		▶	273	249
g. Copies not Distributed (See Instructions to Publishers #4 (page R3))		▶	0	0
h. Total (Sum of 15f and g)		▶	273	249
i. Percent Paid (15c divided by 15f times 100)			96.34%	95.98%

* If you are claiming electronic copies, go to line 16 on page 3. If you are not claiming electronic copies, skip to line 17 on page 3.

PS Form 3526, July 2014 (Page 2 of 4)

16. Electronic Copy Circulation		Average No. Copies Each Issue During Preceding 12 Months	No. Copies of Single Issue Published Nearest to Filing Date
a. Paid Electronic Copies	▶		
b. Total Paid Print Copies (Line 15c) + Paid Electronic Copies (Line 16a)	▶		
c. Total Print Distribution (Line 15f) + Paid Electronic Copies (Line 16a)	▶		
d. Percent Paid (Both Print & Electronic Copies) (16b divided by 16c × 100)	▶		

☒ I certify that 50% of all my distributed copies (electronic and print) are paid above a nominal price.

17. Publication of Statement of Ownership
☒ If the publication is a general publication, publication of this statement is required. Will be printed   ☐ Publication not required.
in the   NOVEMBER 2023   issue of this publication.

18. Signature and Title of Editor, Publisher, Business Manager, or Owner

Malathi Samayan   Date 9/18/2023

Malathi Samayan - Distribution Controller

I certify that all information furnished on this form is true and complete. I understand that anyone who furnishes false or misleading information on this form or who omits material or information requested on the form may be subject to criminal sanctions (including fines and imprisonment) and/or civil sanctions (including civil penalties).

PS Form 3526, July 2014 (Page 3 of 4)   PRIVACY NOTICE: See our privacy policy on www.usps.com

Moving?

Make sure your subscription moves with you!

To notify us of your new address, find your **Clinics Account Number** (located on your mailing label above your name), and contact customer service at:

Email: journalscustomerservice-usa@elsevier.com

800-654-2452 (subscribers in the U.S. & Canada)
314-447-8871 (subscribers outside of the U.S. & Canada)

Fax number: 314-447-8029

Elsevier Health Sciences Division
Subscription Customer Service
3251 Riverport Lane
Maryland Heights, MO 63043

*To ensure uninterrupted delivery of your subscription, please notify us at least 4 weeks in advance of move.

Printed and bound by CPI Group (UK) Ltd, Croydon, CR0 4YY

03/10/2024

01040468-0019